Human Factors in Air Transport

Erik Seedhouse
Anthony Brickhouse
Kimberly Szathmary
E. David Williams

Human Factors in Air Transport

Understanding Behavior and Performance in Aviation

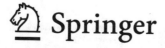 Springer

Erik Seedhouse
Embry-Riddle Aeronautical University
Daytona Beach, FL, USA

Anthony Brickhouse
Embry–Riddle Aeronautical University
Daytona Beach, FL, USA

Kimberly Szathmary
Embry–Riddle Aeronautical University
Daytona Beach, FL, USA

E. David Williams
Embry–Riddle Aeronautical University
Daytona Beach, FL, USA

ISBN 978-3-030-13850-9   ISBN 978-3-030-13848-6   (eBook)
https://doi.org/10.1007/978-3-030-13848-6

This Springer imprint is published by the registered company Springer Nature Switzerland AG.
The registered company address is: Gewerbestrasse 11, 6330 Cham, Switzerland

Contents

About the Authors

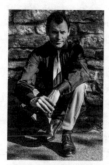

Erik Seedhouse

is a Professor in Spaceflight Operations and Human Factors Aviation Safety at Embry-Riddle Aeronautical University. He has extensive practical and theoretical experience in many of the subjects in this book. After completing his first degree, he joined the 2nd Battalion, the Parachute Regiment. During his time in the "Paras," he spent 6 months in Belize, where he was trained in the art of jungle warfare. Later, he spent several months learning the intricacies of desert warfare in Cyprus. He made more than 30 jumps from a Lockheed C-130 Hercules aircraft, performed more than helicopter 200 abseils, and fired more light anti-tank weapons than he cares to remember!

Upon returning to the academia, he embarked upon a Master's degree supported by winning prize money in 100-km running races. After placing third in the World 100 km Championships in 1992, he turned to ultradistance triathlons, winning the World Endurance Triathlon Championships in 1995 and 1996. For good measure, he won the World Double Ironman Championships in 1995 and the infamous Decatriathlon, an event requiring competitors to swim 38 km, cycle 1800 km, and run 422 km—nonstop!

In 1996, he pursued his Ph.D. at the German Space Agency's Institute for Space Medicine. While studying, he found time to win Ultraman Hawaii and the European Ultraman Championships as well as complete the Race Across America. Due to his success as the world's leading ultradistance triathlete, he was featured in dozens of magazine and television interviews. In 1997, *GQ* magazine named him the "Fittest Man in the World."

In 1999, he took a research job at Simon Fraser University. In 2005, he worked as an Astronaut Training Consultant for Bigelow Aerospace. Between 2008 and 2013, he served as Director of Canada's manned centrifuge and hypobaric operations. In 2009, he was one of the final 30 candidates in the Canadian Space Agency's Astronaut Recruitment Campaign. He has a dream job as a Professor at Embry-Riddle Aeronautical University in Daytona Beach, Florida. He holds a pilot's license and, in his spare time, works as an Astronaut Instructor for Project PoSSUM, an occasional film consultant to Hollywood, a professional speaker, a triathlon coach, and an author. He also serves as a consultant to myriad television productions. This textbook, for which he wrote ▶ Chaps. 1, 2, 3, 4, 7, and 9 and contributed to ▶ Chaps. 5, 6, 8, and 10, is his 28th publication. When not enjoying the sun and rocket launches on Florida's Space Coast with his fiancée, Alice, he divides his time between his second home in Sandefjord and Waikoloa.

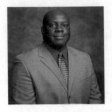

Anthony Brickhouse

is an Associate Professor assigned to the Department of Applied Aviation Sciences in the College of Aviation at the Daytona Beach Campus of Embry-Riddle Aeronautical University. Before joining the faculty of ERAU, he served as the Assistant Aviation Safety Program Manager for the Daytona Beach Campus. Before joining the aviation safety staff at ERAU, he was assigned to the Vehicle Performance Division of the Office of Research and Engineering at the National Transportation Safety Board (NTSB) in Washington, DC. During the span of his career, he has investigated numerous aircraft accidents and safety events. Since entering academia, he has been involved in research surrounding Flight Operations Quality Assurance (FOQA), airport ground safety, the use of flight recorders in accident investigation, and the mental health aspects of accident investigation.

He holds a Bachelor of Science degree in Aerospace Engineering (spacecraft design) with minors in mathematics/aviation safety and a Master of Science degree in Aeronautical Science with a specialization in Aviation/Aerospace Safety Systems. He completed doctoral coursework at the Fischler School of Education and Human Services at Nova Southeastern University, with a focus on higher education leadership in aviation and conflict resolution. He is a Professional Member of the American Society of Safety Professionals (ASSP) and is a Full Member of the International Society of Air Safety Investigators (ISASI), serving on their General Aviation Safety and Unmanned Aircraft Systems Working Groups. He is also the International Coordinator of Student Outreach and Mentoring for ISASI. Anthony is the primary contributor to ▶ Chap. 1 of this book.

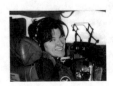

Kimberly Szathmary

is an Assistant Professor of Aerospace Safety in the Department of Applied Aviation Sciences, College of Aviation, at Embry-Riddle Aeronautical University's Daytona Beach Campus, and Manager of the University's new Flight Data Analysis Lab. She currently teaches introductory aerospace safety, human factors, safety program management, and digital safety data analysis courses in the classroom and has also taught via the online and EagleVision (synchronous) modalities for the University's Worldwide Campus. She previously taught and developed award-winning faculty development series course worldwide. She earned a Ph.D. in International Business, Management, and Aeronautical Science in 2014 at Northcentral University, Prescott, AZ, while researching Airline Service Quality and earned a Master of Aeronautical Science in 1995 from Embry-

Riddle. She is a 1984 graduate of Valdosta State University, Valdosta, GA. Her current research interests include predictive flight modeling, data visualization, unmanned systems safety, cockpit video, and using flight data analysis to detect precursors to loss of control inflight.

She is also involved in research in unmanned systems and their integration into the National Airspace System and is a contributor to books such as this one for which she wrote most of ▶ Chaps. 5 and 10. She is a retired US Air Force Pilot, having flown the T-37, T-38, C-141B, and C-17A and was a Senior Supervisor of Flying, which entailed direct control of as many as 40 heavy aircraft in missions ranging from airdrop, air refueling, low-level maneuvering, instrument and visual flight, and assault landings. She also holds all equivalent FAA flight and instructor certificates. Her son, Luke, is an Aerospace Engineering Major at Embry-Riddle Aeronautical University's Daytona Beach Campus.

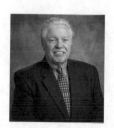

E. David Williams

is an Assistant Professor of Aeronautical and Occupational Safety in the College of Aviation at Embry-Riddle Aeronautical University in Daytona Beach, Florida. He teaches aviation safety and airport operations to both undergraduate and graduate classes. He is an experienced pilot with commercial, multiengine, and instrument flight ratings. His flying experience provided him with particular insight into the challenges faced by pilots described in ▶ Chap. 6, of which he was the primary author. Before joining ERAU, he was engaged as a Risk Manager and Loss Control Specialist in the insurance industry. Prior to this, he was the Executive Director of the Golden Triangle Regional Airport in Columbus, MS, and served as the Chairman of the Anniston, AL Airport Commission. He is a former US Air Force Combat Pilot and served in Vietnam. He also holds the profession designations of Associate in Risk Management (ARM) and the Accredited Advisor in Insurance (AAI) from the American Institute for Chartered Property and Casualty Underwriters.

Human Factors: An Introduction

© Springer Nature Switzerland AG 2020
E. Seedhouse et al., *Human Factors in Air Transport*,
https://doi.org/10.1007/978-3-030-13848-6_1

1

Learning Objectives
After completing this chapter, you should be able to
— Describe the work of Frank and Lillian Gilbreth in the development of human factors
— Describe the events leading up to the 1977 Tenerife disaster
— List the Dirty Dozen
— Describe the context of each Dirty Dozen factor as it applies to aviation
— Explain what caused the Columbia accident
— Describe the work of Paul Fitts
— List the key events in the evolution of human factors in the prewar and postwar eras
— Describe some of the problems that occurred in the transition from traditional cockpits to glass cockpits
— Describe the application of the SHEL model in the context of human factors and error
— Distinguish between Software, Hardware, Environment and Liveware and provide an example of each in the aviation environment

1.1 Human Factors

What do we mean by "Human Factors"? The term has been around for several decades now, having been coined by British psychologist Hywel Murrell in 1949. It describes a multidisciplinary science that encompasses psychology, engineering, industrial design, statistics, human performance, operations research and anthropometry. It is a science that seeks to understand the parameters of human performance and to apply this understanding to the design, development and operation of systems such as aircraft. As you can imagine, the application of human factors is no easy task given its multifaceted structure. In short, there is no simple fix in the realm of human factors because it is difficult to understand exactly how people will be affected by certain conditions under a range of circumstances. We'll get into how this is achieved in this book, but first, some backstory.

1.1.1 Frank and Lillian Gilbreth

The origins of today's human factors can be traced back to the work of Frank (◘ Fig. 1.1) and Lillian Gilbreth, two industrial engineers who worked to try to reduce human error in medicine in the 1900s. One of their innovations was to introduce the use of "call backs" in the operating room. For example, the surgeon says "forceps" and the assistant repeats "forceps" and then hands the instrument to the surgeon. This human factors innovation is termed the *challenge-response system*. It is a simple but very effective system, because by speaking out loud, the surgeon is given the opportunity to correct if the particular instrument requested is not the right tool. The challenge-response system has long been used as a verbal protocol in aviation, with pilots required to read back instructions and clearances given by air traffic control (ATC).

At about the same time that the Gilbreths were pioneering their human factors work in medicine, the Wright Brothers (◘ Fig. 1.2) were working on aviation challenges at Kill Devil Hills, near Kitty Hawk, North Carolina. Some of these challenges included developing human interactive controls for aircraft pitch, roll and yaw. These controls were put to the test when the brothers made a series of powered flights at Kitty Hawk on December

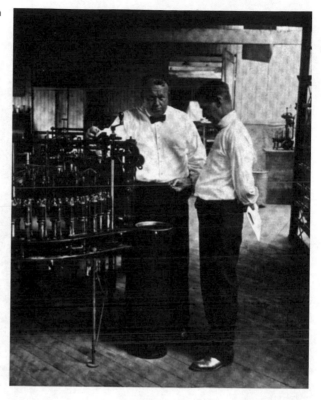

□ Fig. 1.1 Frank Gilbreth. Open source image

17, 1903. The brothers, made famous by these pioneering flights, were the first to apply human factors (not recognized as a science back in those days) not only in the development of flight controls but also in the development of systems that reduced pilot workload, such as inflight control of power and an angle of attack sensor. They later went on to develop a flight simulator and patented many flight control systems [1].

1.1.2 World War I – World War II

» It should be possible to eliminate a large proportion of so-called "pilot-error" accidents by designing equipment in accordance with human requirements

- Opening quote from *Analysis of factors contributing to 460 'pilot-error' experiences in operating aircraft controls*. Published by Fitts and Jones [2]

The evolution of human factors continued with the onset of World War I, which required that sophisticated equipment be developed and that personnel be trained in the operation of said equipment. This requirement demanded an understanding of human capabilities and also human psychology, two important elements of the science of human factors [3, 4]. For example, those involved in the design of the aircraft needed to understand the effects of altitude and G-forces (□ Fig. 1.3) on the pilot. They also needed to know how best to position the controls and displays to ensure optimum performance when flying.

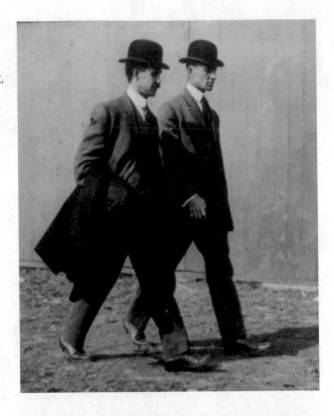

Fig. 1.2 Wright brothers at the Belmont Park Aviation Meet in 1910. Credit: Library of Congress, Prints and Photographs Division, Washington, DC, 20540, USA

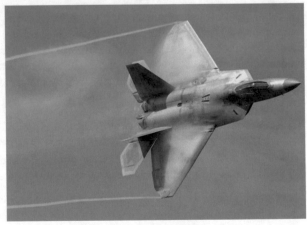

Fig. 1.3 A US Air Force F-22 Raptor piloted by a member of the Air Combat Command F-22 Demonstration Team performs aerial maneuvers during the Arctic Thunder Open House at Joint Base Elmendorf-Richardson, Alaska. Credit: USAF/Photo by Alejandro Pena

One of the outcomes of all this work was the establishment of two aeronautical laboratories at the end of World War I: one at Brooks Air Force Base in Texas, and one at Wright Field near Dayton in Ohio. World War II also served as a catalyst, again spurring work in human factors. Since World War I, aviation systems had evolved at a rapid rate of knots, and by the late 1930s there was a much greater requirement to consider human limitations and not exceed human capabilities.

Meeting this challenge took time and required a significant amount of research. One standout study in this realm was conducted by Fitts and Jones (1947), who analyzed the most effective configuration of controls and dials in the aircraft control panel. To develop their ideal control panel layout, Fitts and Jones examined features of World War II aircraft and analyzed how these features influenced how pilots made errors. For example, pilots would occasionally mistake the gear handles for the flap handles, because not only did these handles look alike, but they were also co-located. On other occasions, pilots might mis-select the throttle and propeller controls because the position of these controls was not consistent across types of aircraft. In the course of their systematic investigations, Fitts and Jones gained an understanding of pilot error and how such errors were systematically linked to features on the control panel. They also learned that errors made more sense once human factors specialists understood the features that pilots interacted with. This last insight was revelatory, forming the underlying basis of what human factors boils down to: that by *re-designing* and *re-building* systems, it is possible to understand why people do what they do and how such systems influence their actions.

1.1.3 The Cold War

The two decades following the end of World War II was a busy time in the development of human factors, thanks in part to the Cold War (◻ Fig. 1.4), which drove much of the military-sponsored research. Military research laboratories developed during this period included the Army's Human Engineering Laboratory, the Air Force's Air Force Personnel and Training Research Center and the Navy's Naval Electronics Laboratory. On the civilian side, the University of Illinois established the Aviation Psychology Laboratory, and Ohio State University founded the Laboratory of Aviation Psychology. In 1957, the Human Factors Society was formed in the US. The society, which today has 4,500 members, has since been rebranded as the Human Factors and Ergonomics Society.

» This basic principle of "human engineering" is not new …. although it has been consistently neglected, largely because engineers concerned with the development of the machine and scientists concerned with the individual who is to operate the machine have worked in almost complete isolation with each other. The resulting disregard of sensory and physiological handicaps; of fundamental principles of perception; of basic patterns of motor coordination; of human limitations in the integration of complex responses has at times led to the production of mechanical monstrosities which tax the capabilities of human operators and hinder the integration of man and machine into a system designed for the most effective accomplishment of designated task.

- Excerpt from the Fitts report, quoting Morris Viteles, the Chairman of the Committee on Aviation Psychology

One of the primary research areas in the Cold War era was on the subject of fatigue and disorientation. One of those leading the charge was the aforementioned Fitts, now a Lt Col [2], who headed an aviation psychology research team at White Field, Ohio. In

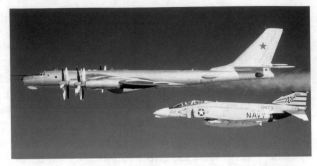

□ Fig. 1.4   United States Navy F-4 Phantom II intercepts a Soviet Tupolev Tu-95 D aircraft in the Cold War. Credit: National Archives and Records Administration

1951, the team presented an author report that identified several key human factor issues in aviation. The report (see above quote), which simply became known as the Fitts Report, summarised key human factors findings of several decades and highlighted a number of challenges that needed to be addressed. These challenges included defining the role of humans in the air traffic system, measuring human performance and behavior, assessing information processing capacity of pilots and controllers, and categorizing tasks that exceeded human capacity [5].

In the same era that Fitts and his team were researching human factors problems, the aviation industry witnessed an explosion in air travel. Unfortunately, the infrastructure was ill-equipped to deal with the increase in traffic. While radar had been developed in the 1940s, it wasn't yet part of civilian air traffic control. Instead, aircraft were monitored using flight status boards, which were not up to the task of coping with the sudden spike in air traffic. The primitiveness of the system was highlighted on June 30, 1956, when a United Airlines Douglas DC-7 collided with a Trans World Airlines Lockheed L-1049 Super Constellation in the Grand Canyon. The collision killed all 128 on board the aircraft—the first time in commercial aviation that an aviation incident had killed more than 100 people. The crash led to significant changes in the control of flights, including the required use of radar to monitor traffic.

1.1.4   1960s and 1970s

The 1960s witnessed more of the same growth in the aviation industry, which not only necessitated rapid development in infrastructure but also a reassessment of how pilots flew the new aircraft that were being introduced. It was in this decade that aircraft such as the Boeing 727, 737 and 747 were developed, and these aircraft featured several new technologies that required a recalibration of the pilot's role (□ Fig. 1.5). The concern was that pilot training was not keeping pace with the new technology being introduced. This worry was highlighted by multiple high-profile accidents in the 1970s, renewing focus on aviation human factors research. One such accident occurred on December 29, 1972, when an Eastern Airlines Lockheed L-1011 TriStar crashed in the Florida Everglades and resulted in the loss of 101 passengers and crew. The cause? The crew had been so fixated on a burned-out landing gear that they hadn't noticed the aircraft losing altitude!

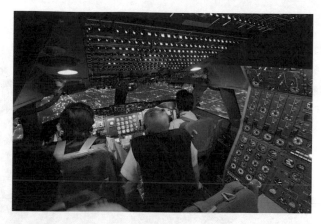

Fig. 1.5 An early-production 747 cockpit, located on the upper deck. Credit: Shahram Sharifi

» …the failure of the flight crew to monitor the flight instruments during the final four minutes of flight, and to detect an unexpected descent soon enough to prevent impact with the ground. Preoccupation with a malfunction of the nose landing gear position indicating system distracted the crew's attention from the instruments and allowed the descent to go unnoticed.

- Excerpt from the US National Transportation Safety Board report AAR-73/14 citing the cause of the Eastern Airlines crash as pilot error

After the Eastern Airlines disaster, the NTSB recommended changes to prevent similar accidents. One of these changes was to the altitude warning system. At the time of the Eastern Airlines disaster, the altitude warning system gave an audible and visual indication below 2,500 feet. The NTSB changed this indication to a continuous flash. It wasn't a ground breaking change, but it was move in the right direction.

Five years later, the issue of human factors was highlighted in the worst possible way in the Canary Islands. On March 27, 1977, a KLM Boeing 747 and a Pan Am Boeing 747 were preparing for takeoff at Los Rodeos Airport in Tenerife (Aside). Due to a series of human factors errors, the two aircraft collided, resulting in the deaths of 583 people. It was—and still is—the deadliest accident in aviation history (☐ Fig. 1.6).

Aside

Tenerife

On that fateful day in March 1977, Gran Canaria International Airport had been closed due to a bombing. This incident caused several aircraft to be diverted to Los Rodeos, including the KLM and Pan Am Boeing 747s. Tenerife's airport was a regional airport with just a single runway and a few narrow taxiways. This meant that the larger aircraft that had been diverted from Gran Canaria had to park on these taxiways, which in turn meant there was no room for taxiing. The taxiways became so clogged with traffic that the only way for aircraft to depart was to backtrack on the runway. After a lengthy wait, Gran Canaria Airport was reopened and the green light was given for the diverted aircraft to begin preparing for departure. The Pan Am 747 was ready for departure but was unable to take off because it was blocked by the KLM aircraft, which was refueling. By the time refueling had been completed, the weather had taken a turn for the worse, with low clouds and fog descending on the airport.

1

When the KLM aircraft had at last been given taxi clearance, the pilots couldn't see the tower. The KLM 747 was cleared to enter the runway, taxi to the end of the runway and then execute a 180° turn in preparation for takeoff. As the KLM 747 was taxiing to the end of the runway, the Pan Am 747 was given the go ahead to taxi and to follow the KLM 747. It was then instructed to follow the KLM 747, vacate the runway by taking the third taxiway to the left and use a parallel taxiway. Unfortunately, the Pan Am crew did not understand the instructions of the controller and were unsure if they had been instructed to take the first or third exit. As both aircraft continued to taxi, the weather deteriorated even more, limiting visual range to just 1,000 feet. The Pan Am crew, concerned about unclear instructions given to them by the controller, requested clarification on which taxiway to take. The controller responded by instructing Pan Am as follows: "The third one, sir; one, two, three; third, third one".

Armed with this information, the Pan Am 747 proceeded to taxi as instructed, but appeared to still be unsure of their position due to the inclement weather. Meanwhile, the KLM crew believed it had been cleared for takeoff and thought the Pan Am 747 had taken off. Thus thinking the runway was clear, the KLM captain applied full power. Seconds later the Pan Am crew saw the KLM 747's landing lights approaching at a very rapid rate of knots and, in a last-ditch attempt to save the day, applied full power to make a left turn that the crew hoped would avoid the inevitable. At that moment the KLM captain saw the Pan Am 747 and made the decision to rotate early, as it was far too late to apply the brakes. This maneuver caused the KLM's tail to drag along the ground for 70 feet before impacting the top of the Pan Am 747 at approximately 140 knots. The KLM 747 stalled and crashed a short distance away. Since it had just refueled, it rapidly became a fireball. Both aircraft were destroyed.

- Source: Official Joint Report, KLM-Pan AM 12 July 1978

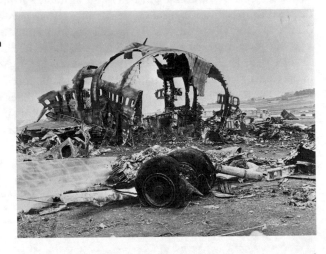

◻ **Fig. 1.6**   Wreckage on the runway of Los Rodeos after the Tenerife airport disaster of March 27, 1977. Credit: Dutch National Archives

The Tenerife disaster catalyzed the industry to make significant changes to international airlines regulations, one of which was to make English the common working aviation language. But language wasn't the only human factors deficiency at the time, as became evident in an accident that echoed the Eastern Airlines accident. On December 28, 1978, a United Airlines DC-8 crashed in a Portland residential area. The cause: the aircraft had run out of fuel, which was a surprise given that the aircraft had had more than enough fuel for the flight. The crew had noticed some strange noises when lowering the landing gear. Then, the landing gear indicator malfunctioned. At this point, with the gear down and locked, the crew should have made a trouble-free landing, but instead they became fixated on trying to diagnose the fault—so fixated that the aircraft crashed to due fuel exhaustion.

» The Safety Board believes that this accident exemplifies a recurring problem—a breakdown in cockpit management and teamwork during a situation involving malfunctions of aircraft systems in flight… Therefore, the Safety Board can only conclude that the flight crew failed to relate the fuel remaining and the rate of fuel flow to the time and distance from the airport, because their attention was directed almost entirely toward diagnosing the landing gear problem.

- Source: NTSB AAR-79/07

The NTSB continued in its report to ensure that "their flight crews are indoctrinated in principles of flight deck resource management, with particular emphasis on the merits of participative management for captains and assertiveness training for other cockpit crewmembers". The United Airlines flight was the catalyst for the birth of formal crew resource management (a term coined by NASA psychologist John Lauber), initially known as cockpit resource management or CRM. Unsurprisingly, United Airlines became the first adopter (in 1981), but many airlines quickly followed. Helping push the CRM initiative along was NASA, which sponsored a 1979 workshop called Resource Management on the Flight Deck. The workshop was largely responsible for many airlines kick-starting their own CRM training (◘ Fig. 1.7). The basic precept for CRM was to dilute the authoritarian culture in the cockpit and encourage copilots to at least ask questions if they observed the captain making a mistake.

In many ways, CRM was a pathfinder ideology that improved situational awareness, enhanced leadership training, improved decision-making and led to a more flexible cockpit environment. Not surprisingly, it is now practiced by all airlines, not only in the realm of cockpit operations but also in areas such as air traffic control and aviation maintenance (◘ Fig. 1.8).

◘ **Fig. 1.7** Crew resource management training in a Royal Air Force Nimrod aircraft. Credit: RAF (Open Government License)/ Photo: SAC Brown RAF/MOD

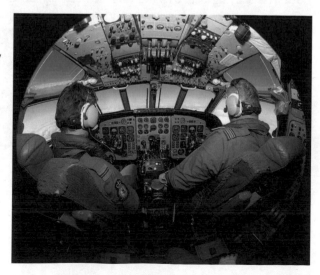

1

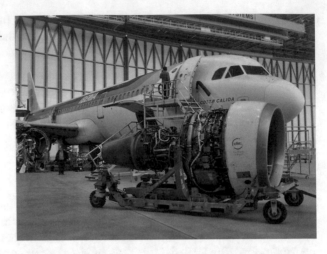

◘ **Fig. 1.8**   An Airbus 321 from Iberia having its CFM56 changed. Credit: Curimedia – Airbus A321-211Iberia EC-IGK

1.1.5 1980s

The 1980s witnessed a dramatic increase in automation that should have brought about a reduction in workload and increased safety. For the most part it did, but as with any introduction of automation, there were pitfalls. For example, the newly introduced glass cockpits were implicated in a number of human factors accidents. The problem affected the older crews more than the younger crews, simply because the older crews had spent so much more time using the traditional instruments and therefore found the transition to glass instruments more demanding. Another aspect of the transition was the change in crew coordination, which became more complex due to the introduction of the flight management computer (FMC) and the flight management system (FMS). Many of the incidents at the time these systems were being introduced occurred as a result of entering incorrect information into the FMS (Aside). Other incidents were attributed to forgetting basic flying skills as pilots became over-dependent on the automation.

Aside

American Airlines Flight
On December 20, 1995, an American Airlines Boeing 757 crashed into a mountain in Columbia. The aircraft, which had been en-route from Miami to Cali, Columbia, featured a FMS. It was while reprogramming this system that the crew made an error that ultimately led to the crash.

In 1995, Cali ATC required approaching aircraft to navigate using radio beacons to avoid the mountainous terrain. The 757's FMS had the locations of these beacons in its database, and navigation should not have

been a problem. Unfortunately, the crew erased all the waypoints identifying the beacons while reprogramming the FMS! When asked by flight controllers to report over one of the waypoints, the crew had to resort to paper charts to locate the waypoint. This took so much time that when the chart had finally been located, the aircraft had flown past the waypoint. In desperation, the crew attempted to reprogram the waypoints but entered the incorrect information, which directed the aircraft towards the 3,000-meter mountain.

How could the American Airlines accident have been avoided? Well, the crew could have been better trained in the use of automation, and they could have better distributed the workload across the crew. Human factors yet again.

Another aid that helps pilots with automation is *flight envelope protection*, an initiative developed by Airbus that prevents crews from making control inputs that exceed structural limits. It is essentially a human error-limiting device. The problem with humans is that we tend to be extraordinarily creative when it comes to finding new ways in which to commit errors. This means that it is very difficult to design an error-proof system—all the best envelope protections in the world can't protect a confused and befuddled crew. Consider the case of the China Airlines Airbus accident that occurred on April 26, 1994. On that date, China Airlines Flight B1816 took off from Taipei Airport en-route for Nagoya. On its ILS approach to Nagoya's Runway 34, the flight officer accidently activated the GO lever, which altered the Flight Director to Go Around mode. This resulted in a thrust increase that in turn caused the aircraft to deviate from its flight path and enter an out-of-trim configuration. The crew, unaware of the inadvertent change of mode, continued the approach as the angle of attack increased. Too late, the crew noticed the high pitch angle. The aircraft crashed, killing 264 passengers and crew.

How, in the face of all this automation, fail-safes and envelope protections, could such an accident have occurred? Well, the Takeoff/Go around switch, as its name implies, has two modes: Takeoff and Go around. The modes are specific to the flight phase. So, on approach, the autopilot will be set to approach mode, which means if it is pressed it will change to Go around mode and vice versa. On Boeing aircraft, these modes are activated by pressing a switch near the throttle levers, whereas on an Airbus, these modes are activated by moving the thrust levers forward. So, the way the Airbus controls are configured means that the autopilot cannot be disengaged by pressing the Takeoff/Go around switch. Instead, in the Airbus way of doing things, this action causes the aircraft to stop following the ILS and perform the go around automatically. If it seems confusing, it is, and the accident report highlighted a number of points related to the confusing man-machine interface, some of which are not always intuitive. Not only that, but different aircraft manufacturers have different approaches in designing flight safety automation—a lack of standardization that can be confusing and lead to sometimes disastrous consequences.

1.2 The Dirty Dozen

A significant number of maintenance-related aviation accidents occurred in the 1980 and 1990s. This spate of incidents prompted Transport Canada to launch an investigation, the outcome of which was the identification of 12 human factors that degrade human performance. This group of human factors (see below), which is known as the *Dirty Dozen*, has since been adopted by the aviation industry (◘ Fig. 1.9 and Appendix I). While the list was created based on the research conducted on maintenance incidents, each factor can be applied to aviation in general.

◘ Fig. 1.9 The Dirty Dozen.
Credit: FAA

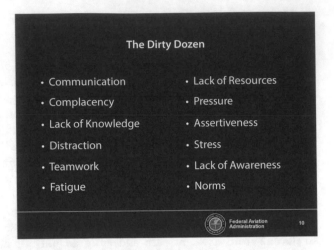

1.2.1 Lack of Communication

Imprecise communication, especially improper procedures, can be the catalyst for a potential error chain. For example, in the AMT world, it is critical that information is exchanged from one technician to another (during shift changes for example). It is also critical that procedures be conducted *exactly* according to approved instructions. And, when the work has been completed, that work must be reviewed, discussed and signed off—again, in accordance with regulations.

1.2.2 Complacency

This particular human factor is one that develops over time. Employees, whether they be AMTs or pilots, gain knowledge and satisfaction in a job that is performed proficiently. In some cases, this sense of proficiency can lapse into false confidence. For example, a simple check that has been performed hundreds of times before without finding a fault may one day be a check that is skipped because it may be judged as unimportant. Another aspect of complacency may occur in task repetition. Routine checks that must be performed repetitively may cause an employee's mind to wander, with the result that critical steps are omitted.

1.2.3 Lack of Knowledge

In the aviation world, a lack of knowledge can have catastrophic consequences. It is a standard-driven industry that demands each person perform to specific standards specified in specialized instructions. These standards and instructions have been developed based on knowledge gleaned from the operation of the equipment. Needless to say, a knowledge gap in any procedure is a recipe for a less than positive outcome.

1.2.4 **Distraction**

Distraction can result in disruption. In the AMT world, it is estimated that distraction causes 15% of all maintenance errors. Fifteen percent! So what causes distraction? Well, distraction can be mental, and there is perhaps no more distracting a technological device than the cellphone. While there has been no reported incident of a texting aviation technician causing an accident, the cellphone played a prominent role in a fatal accident in 2011. On August 26, 2011, a Eurocoptor AS350 B2 ran out of fuel in Missouri, killing the pilot, a nurse, paramedic and patient [6]. The probable cause as noted by the NTSB was:

» ...pilot's failure to confirm that the helicopter had adequate fuel on board to complete the mission before making the first departure, his improper decision to continue the mission and make a second departure after he became aware of a critically low fuel level, and his failure to successfully enter an autorotation when the engine lost power due to fuel exhaustion

- Source: NTSB Accident ID: CEN11FA599. NTSB Number: AAR-13-02. NTIS Number: PB2013-104866

Why had the pilot failed to check the fuel level? He had been texting! His inability to separate himself from his cellphone resulted in him failing to complete the preflight inspection and failing to conduct an emergency landing, as noted by the NTSB in the contributing factors section of its report:

» ...the pilot's distracted attention due to personal texting during safety-critical ground and flight operations...Once the pilot made his decision to proceed with this mission nothing was going to deter him from his course, regardless of whether he used a cell phone.

- Source: NTSB Accident ID: CEN11FA599. NTSB Number: AAR-13-02. NTIS Number: PB2013-104866

The report continued to describe the pilot's texting as a "source of distraction and interruptions", citing research that distracting devices such as cellphones "decrease cognitive capacity, reduce the processing of potentially relevant information and can cause information in working memory to be confused or forgotten. These effects degrade performance of complex tasks and increase the likelihood of decision errors".

1.2.5 **Lack of Teamwork**

The aviation industry is all about teamwork, but this human factor element can easily be compromised by personality conflicts, poor communication, lack of coordination and lack of consensus. This factor can also be eroded by individuals in the organization not performing their roles correctly. One weak link and effective teamwork can quickly degrade.

1.2.6 **Fatigue**

Fatigue is deadly and has been cited as a major human factor in all sorts of aviation accidents. Fatigue can be mental, physical and/or emotional and can cause a reduction in alertness,

1

compromised decision-making, increased reaction time, reduced strength, impaired cognitive ability, poor judgement and loss of situational awareness. Preventing fatigue, as we shall see later in this book, is no easy task when working in an industry that never sleeps and when personnel must routinely transit multiple time zones every day. Surprisingly, in an industry that is so heavily regulated, there is no metric for assessing fatigue.

1.2.7 Lack of Resources

Lack of resources equates to lack of supply and support, and without these, one's ability to perform the task at hand is compromised. Similarly, low quality products can affect safety, which is why it is so important to have the right tools for the task. Products do not necessarily have to mean equipment—technical documentation and manuals need to be written correctly and revisions to them maintained.

1.2.8 Pressure

Aviation is an industry with tight schedules, and operating under a tight schedule inevitably means working under pressure. This creates a kind of environment in which one's judgment can become clouded and mistakes can be made. One way to reduce the incidence of mistakes is to implement checks of work done and to bring concerns to the organization's management.

1.2.9 Lack of Assertiveness

This is a term that simply describes your ability to express your opinions and beliefs in a positive and productive manner. Assertiveness should not be mistaken for aggression, and there is sometimes a fine line between the two. Why is this human factor so important? Well, the consequences of lack of assertiveness can ultimately cost lives. Consider the case of Alaska Airlines Flight 261 [7]. This flight was scheduled to fly between Puerto Vallarta, Mexico to Seattle, USA with an intermediate stop in San Francisco, but the MD-83 aircraft crashed a few miles north of Anacapa Island, California, killing all 88 passengers and crew. The NTSB found the culprit to be an inflight failure of the horizontal stabilizer trim system jackscrew assembly's nut threads. This was later identified as a defect in the MD-83 aircraft, but why had such a flaw gone undetected? Well, one human factor was pressure. Before the accident, it was noted that a jackscrew needed to be replaced [8]. But ordering said jackscrew would have delayed the aircraft's departure, so the maintenance log was falsified and the aircraft was pronounced airworthy! The maintenance personnel was aware of the problem but did not speak up, despite knowing what the consequences might be.

1.2.10 Stress

Stress is an integral feature of the world of aviation, but what is stress? There is the spectrum of stressors to consider. This can include physical stressors such as workload, temperature, noise, lighting, work-related issues and financial problems. Stressors can also include physiological contributors such as fatigue, hunger, illness, lack of sleep and poor health. Conflicting schedules, circadian rhythm upset, excessive alcohol use and smoking can also be included in the list of stressors, and each conspires to exert a stressful effect on the individual with the outcome being degradation in performance.

1.2.11 Lack of Awareness

This human factor element is a failure to recognize the consequences of an action or can be simply construed as a lack of vigilance. In the operation of an aircraft, it is normal to perform identical tasks hundreds of times, and it is only human nature to become less vigilant when performing such repetition. To counter this, it is necessary to perform a task as it if it is being performed for the first time.

1.2.12 Norms

Norms are the unwritten rules followed by those in any industry. They are usually developed to resolve ambiguous problems. In this instance, an individual may use another individuals' response as a frame of reference to react to solve the problem. Over time this reaction can become the standard—or norm—and in most cases these norms are fairly benign. A problem arises when these norms become negative or unsafe, in which case they deviate from the standard—for example, by taking shortcuts or not following procedures.

1.2.13 1990s

In the 1990s, the aviation industry witnessed new regulations in Europe that resulted in mandatory categories of flight crew training and controller training. This decade also saw an improvement in flight data recorder analysis and the introduction of Threat and Error Management (TEM), a safety management initiative developed by the University of Texas. The framework for TEM assumes that pilots will make mistakes, and its goal is to ensure safety by training flight crews to detect and respond to off-nominal events. Like Flight Operational Quality Assurance (FOQA), TEM is a proactive approach to threat identification [8]. It comprises three components of threats, errors and undesired aircraft states (UAS). The premise of the model is that mistakes are an everyday part of flying an aircraft, and that these mistakes have the potential to cause undesired aircraft states. The goal of TEM is for the pilot to manage the undesired aircraft states to prevent an undesirable outcome. In the context of TEM, threats are defined (by ICAO) as "events or errors that occur beyond the influence of the flight crew, increase operational complexity, and which must be managed to maintain the margins of safety". Such events might include dealing with mountainous terrain, CRM deficiencies, aircraft malfunctions, or a combination of these. Some of these threats may be anticipated. For example, a pilot can see a thunderstorm approaching on the

□ Table 1.1   Operational threats

Environmental threats	Organisational threats
Weather: thunderstorms, turbulence, icing, wind shear, very high/low temperature	**Operational pressure:** delays late arrivals, equipment changes
ATC: traffic congestion, ATC language difficulty, ATC runway change	**Aircraft:** aircraft malfunction, automation anomaly
Airport: contaminated/short runway, confusing signage, birds	**Cabin:** flight attendant error, cabin distraction, cabin door security
Terrain: high ground slope, lack of references	**Maintenance:** maintenance error

Adapted from ICAO. Under the TEM model. Threats are grouped into those that may occur spontaneously (Environmental) and those that can be controlled (Organisational)

weather radar and brief the passengers accordingly for the consequences, thereby avoiding a more serious event. On the other hand, some threats may be latent and not obvious or observable by the crew, such as an aircraft malfunction or a turn-around deadline. Under the TEM model, the metric used to determine the crew's ability to mitigate and manage threats is to reduce the threat-error linkage and respond to a threat (□ Table 1.1) by implementing effective countermeasures [8].

The second component of the TEM model is error. Errors are defined by ICAO as "actions or inactions by the flight crew that lead to deviations from organizational or flight crew intentions or expectations". The extent to which an error affects safety depends on the flight crew detecting and responding to that error before the error (□ Table 1.2) causes an unsafe state or undesired outcome. This "detection and response" is at the core of the TEM model.

In the TEM model, error classification is based on the interaction of the pilot when the error is made. So, for an error to be classified as a *handling error*, the crew must be interacting with the aircraft, whereas for an error to be classified as a *procedural error*, the crew must make a procedural error when interacting with a checklist for example.

1.2.14   **2000s**

In the 2000s, a greater emphasis was placed on considering groups rather than individuals, and categorizing accidents into those caused by individuals and those caused by organizational action or inaction. One classic—and tragic—example of epic organizational failure was the Columbia Space Shuttle disaster (□ Fig. 1.10) that occurred on February 1, 2003, killing the crew of seven [9]. During launch, a briefcase-sized chunk of foam insulation shed from the External Tank and struck Columbia's left wing. Foam strikes were not unusual, having occurred on numerous Shuttle launches over the years. But after reviewing the damage following Columbia's launch, engineers reckoned the damage was a lot more serious. The engineers then voiced their concerns with NASA managements, but these concerns fell on deaf ears. The engineers

◨ **Table 1.2** Examples of errors

Aircraft handling errors	**Manual handling/flight controls**: vertical/lateral and/or speed deviations, incorrect flaps/speed brakes.
	Automation: incorrect altitude, speed, heading, auto throttle settings, incorrect mode executed
	Systems/radio instruments: incorrect packs, incorrect anti-icing, incorrect altimeter
	Ground navigation: attempting to turn down wrong taxiway/runway, taxi too fast
Procedural errors	**SOPs**: failure to cross-verify automation inputs
	Checklists: wrong challenge and response, items missed, checklist performed late
	Callouts: omitted/incorrect callouts
	Briefings: omitted briefings, items missed
	Documentation: wrong weight and balance, fuel information, ATIS or clearance information
Communication errors	**Crew to external**: missed calls, misinterpretations of instructions, incorrect read-back, wrong clearance
	Pilot-to-pilot: within crew miscommunication or misinterpretation

In the TEM mode, errors are grouped in three categories. Adapted from ICAO

◨ **Fig. 1.10** Space Shuttle Columbia disaster. Credit: NASA

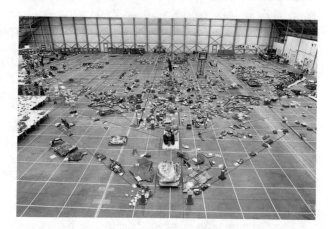

didn't give up and requested imagery of the left wing by a Department of Defence satellite. NASA management refused these requests and actually tried to prevent the DoD from helping the agency. Predictably enough, the Columbia Accident Investigation Board (CAIB) was damning in its indictment of NASA' upper management organization deficiencies and flaws in the agency's decision-making and risk-assessment procedures.

1

Regarding organizational causes, the Board concluded the accident was:

» ... rooted in the Space Shuttle Program's history and culture, including the original compromises that were required to gain approval for the Shuttle, subsequent years of resource constraints, fluctuating priorities, schedule pressures, mischaracterization of the Shuttle as operational rather than developmental, and lack of an agreed national vision for human space flight. Cultural traits and organizational practices detrimental to safety were allowed to develop, including: reliance on past success as a substitute for sound engineering practices..., organizational barriers that prevented effective communication of critical safety information and stifled professional differences of opinion; lack of integrated management across program elements; and the evolution of an informal chain of command and decision-making processes that operated outside the organization's rules.

- Excerpt from the CAIB (p. 9)

The CAIB, while specific to manned spaceflight, nevertheless highlighted several human factors that are involved in accidents [9]. In particular, the findings of the board emphasized the importance of the safety chain and that each link in that chain involves human inputs. Regardless of whether those human inputs are supporting a Shuttle launch or the operation of an aircraft, each link represents an opportunity for an error to occur. Furthermore, the findings of the CAIB accepted that while human error is avoidable, it is manageable.

1.3 Errors and Accidents

On January 8, 1989, British Midland Flight 92, a new Boeing 737-400, was on a scheduled flight from London Heathrow Airport to Belfast Airport [10]. After an emergency landing attempt at East Midlands Airport, 47 of the 126 people onboard were reported dead, and 74 had sustained serious injuries. A series of errors by the flight crew in response to an engine failure caused this accident.

As the flight was climbing through 28,000 feet towards a cruising altitude of 35,000, the #1 Engine (left engine) suffered a broken fan blade. This caused severe vibrations, impacted the air conditioning, and caused smoke to enter the fight deck. The pilots initially didn't know the cause of the problem. Several passengers seated on the left side of the aircraft noticed smoke and sparks coming from the left engine. The plane was being piloted by a 43-year-old Captain and a 39-year-old First Officer. This flight crew had over 16,000 total flight hours combined. Close to 1,000 of those hours were in Boeing 737 aircraft, but only 76 were logged in the new Boeing 737-400 series, the accident aircraft.

The Captain responded by disengaging the autopilot. The pilots then discussed which engine had failed, and there was confusion as to whether it was the right (#2) or left (#1) engine. In older model 737s, the left air conditioning pack used compressor bleed air from the left (#1) engine to supply air to the flight deck. Using the same process, the right (#2) engine supplied air to the cabin. The new 737-400 had a different design, where the #1 engine fed the flight deck and the aft cabin, while the #2 engine fed the forward cabin.

During the investigation, the Captain stated that his perception was that smoke was coming forward from the cabin, leading him to assume the right engine was at fault. The decision was made to secure the right engine, which was the good engine. After doing this, the flight crew could no longer smell smoke and assumed the problem had been addressed correctly. This was not the case. When the autothrottle was disengaged to shut down the right engine, the fuel flow to the left engine was reduced, the damage was reduced, the smoke smell subsided, and the vibrations reduced.

During the approach into the East Midlands Airport, the damaged #1 (left engine) completely failed. Attempts to restart the good #2 (right engine) were unsuccessful. The tail of the aircraft impacted the ground just before crossing the M1 Motorway. The aircraft then bounced over the motorway, crashed into an embankment and broke into three sections. Fortunately, no vehicles were impacted during the crash sequence.

Unlike older 737 models, the bleed air for the cabin air conditioning came from both engines. Several cabin crewmembers and passengers all saw the damaged left engine, but this critical information was never passed along to the flight crew. While running an important component of the emergency checklist, the pilots were interrupted by an ATC transmission. The flight crew never resumed the checklist after this moment. Another area to address involved the vibration indicators. The vibration indicators on the new 737-400 were smaller than on previous models. Also, they were now digital, with LED needles around the outside of the dial instead of analog needles on the inside of the dial. Finally, the flight crew had not received any simulator training on the new 737-400.

Connecting the dots, it is clear how several errors came together to cause a tragedy. If any of these individual errors had not occurred, there is a possibility this accident could have been avoided. Humans are prone to make errors, and this tendency increases during complex tasks. British Midland Flight 92 is a prime example of the importance of human factors and dissecting events to learn as much as possible and to hopefully prevent future occurrences.

1.4 The SHEL Model

How are errors made? How and why do accidents happen? These are two basic questions that continue to plague the safety professionals of today. In most situations, the answers to these questions have a connection to the all-important human element. When safety events or accidents occur, it is imperative that causal factors be determined so that in the end, preventative steps can be taken. One explanation that sought to explain how accidents occurred was dubbed the Single Causation Theory. This early theory held that all accidents and safety events were caused by a singular factor. Many people bought into this belief because of how simple it was to peg one factor as the cause. Not much investigating was done, and a popular cause of accidents became pilot error. Was it really just a mistake the flight crew made, or were there deeper issues?

As safety progressed, the community began to embrace the Multiple Causation Theory, which held that accidents and safety events were caused by several different factors that aligned. This theory continues to be supported by the safety community today. Safety is not enhanced when an investigation focuses on one individual and a

1

sometimes isolated cause. Our systems of today are diverse, with ample connections. When an accident or safety event occurs, it is the job of the safety professional to investigate and determine causal factors.

There are numerous "human-focused" models that guide investigations into the causal factors of accidents. One such model is called the SHEL Model [11–13]. The letters represent Software, Hardware, Environment, and Liveware. As you can see from the model, the blocks naturally fit together. When an accident or safety event occurs, there is a breakdown in one of the areas or relationships. Take special note of the placement of Liveware (human) at the center. The SHEL Model allows one to study the various relationships/interactions between different components to hopefully identify accident causing/inducing failures.

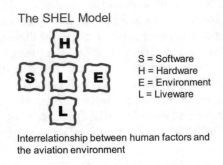

The SHEL Model

S = Software
H = Hardware
E = Environment
L = Liveware

Interrelationship between human factors and the aviation environment

- **Liveware**

At the core of the model is the human, arguably the most important component of any system. In order for any system to work properly, there must be coordinated interactions with the humans involved. It could be argued that humans by their nature are hard to predict and error prone. Because of this, understanding the connection of the Liveware to the other components is imperative.

- **Software – Liveware**

This interaction is focused on the human's interaction with procedures, checklists, training, symbology, and other non-physical aspects of the system.

- **Hardware – Liveware**

This interaction is focused on the human's interaction with machines and equipment. Obviously, as our systems continually become more advanced, this interaction will become even more critical to safe operations.

- **Environment – Liveware**

Each spring in the United States, we experience a spike in general aviation accidents associated with thunderstorms. Pilots for various reasons get too close to convective activity, some with fatal consequences. This interaction is focused on the human's interaction with their operating condition. Also included in this interaction are factors such as fatigue, sleep patterns, and circadian dysynchronization. This interface was one of the earliest ones discovered by the aviation pioneers flying in the early 1900s.

- **Liveware – Liveware**

"See something, say something" is a mantra that plays out in today's aviation world. Thanks to programs such as Crew Resource Management (CRM) and others, everyone involved in the operation of a flight has a role in safety. This interaction is focused on leadership, crew cooperation, personalities, communication and crew gradient. Though the Captain (Commander) has ultimate authority, the First Officer and Cabin Crewmembers should have a significantly important voice as well.

- **Culture – Liveware**

In recent years, the new component of *culture* has been added to the SHEL Model. This addition brings the model into the Safety Management Systems world that aviation/ aerospace operates in. Safety Culture should be at the core of any operation. The culture addition is two-pronged. It includes safety culture as well as the physical culture of the humans in the system. These are two critical considerations when it comes to overall safety and understanding why accidents and safety events occur.

1.5 Summary

As the science of human factors has developed over the years, it has been increasingly applied to the myriad specialties within the aviation arena. Thanks to the continuing work of human factors engineers and scientists, it is possible to apply theories and models that help explain accidents, loss of situational awareness and a host of other issues that may compromise safety in aviation.

> **Key Terms**
> **AMT** - Air Maintenance Technician
> **ATC** - Air Traffic Control
> **CAIB** - Columbia Accident Investigation Board
> **CRM** - Crew Resource Management
> **FMC** - Flight Management Computer
> **FMS** - Flight Management System
> **FOQA** - Flight Operational Quality Assurance
> **ILS** - Instrument Lighting System
> **TEM** - Threat and Error Management
> **UAS** - Undesired Aircraft States

1

Review Questions
1. What is meant by Lack of Awareness in the context of the Dirty Dozen?
2. What were the findings of the CAIB?
3. What was the cause of the Alaska Airlines flight 261?
4. Describe the work of Frank and Lillian Gilbreth in the development of human factors
5. Describe the Multiple Causation Theory
6. Why is the addition of "Culture" to the SHEL Model so significant?
7. What were some key factors in the British Midland Flight 92 accident?

References

1. Dul, J., Bruder, R., Buckle, P., Carayon, P., Falzon, P., Marras, W.S., Wilson, J.R., van der Doelen, B.: A strategy for human factors/ergonomics: developing the discipline and profession. Ergonomics. **55**, 377–395 (2012)
2. Fitts, P.M., Jones, R.E.: Analysis of factors contributing to 460 "pilot error" experiences in operating aircraft controls. Aero Medical Laboratory, Air Material Command, Wright-Patterson Air Force Base, Dayton, OH (1947)
3. Karwowski, W.: From past to future: building a collective vision for HFES 2020+. Hum. Factors Ergon. Soc. Bull. **49**(11), 1–3 (2006)
4. Meister, D.: The History of Human Factors and Ergonomics. Lawrence Erlbaum Associates, Mahwah, NJ (1999)
5. Fitts, P.M., Jones, R.E.: Psychological aspects of instrument display. Analysis of 270 "pilot-error" experiences in reading and interpreting aircraft instruments (Report No. TSEAA-694-12A). Aero Medical Laboratory, Air Materiel Command, U.S. Air Force, Dayton, OH (1947)
6. NTSB: Crash following loss of engine power due to fuel exhaustion; Air Methods Corporation; Euro-copter AS350 B2, N352LN; Near Mosby, MO; August 26, 2011, Aircraft Accident Report NTSB/AAR-13/02, 9 Apr 2013
7. NTSB: Aircraft accident incident report. Loss of Control and Impact with Pacific Ocean Alaska Airlines Flight 261 McDonnell Douglas MD-83, N963AS About 2.7 Miles North of Anacapa Island, CA, January 31, 2000. National Transportation Safety Board, Washington, DC (2002)
8. O'Brien, T.G., Meister, D.: Human factors testing and evaluation: an historical perspective. In: Charlton, S.G., O'Brien, T.G. (eds.) Handbook of Human Factors Testing and Evaluation, pp. 5–20. Lawrence Erlbaum Associates, Mahwah, NJ (2001)
9. Columbia Accident Investigation Board: https://history.nasa.gov/columbia/CAIB.html
10. UK Department of Transport, Air Accidents Investigation Branch, AAR4/1990
11. Australian Government, Civil Aviation Safety Authority: Safety Management Systems for Aviation: A Practical Guide, 2nd edn. Civil Aviation Safety Authority, Canberra, Australia (2014)
12. Cusick, S.K., Cortes, A.I., Rodrigues, C.C.: Commercial Aviation Safety, 6th edn. McGraw-Hill, New York, NY (2017)
13. Hawkins, F.H.: Human Factors in Flight, 2nd edn. Ashgate, Brookfield, VT (1993)

Suggested Reading
Hawkins, F.H.: Human Factors in Flight, 2nd edn. Ashgate, Brookfield, VT (1993)
Meister, D.: The History of Human Factors and Ergonomics. Lawrence Erlbaum Associates, Mahwah, NJ (1999)

Fatigue

© Springer Nature Switzerland AG 2020
E. Seedhouse et al., *Human Factors in Air Transport*,
https://doi.org/10.1007/978-3-030-13848-6_2

2

Learning Objectives

After completing this chapter, you should be able to

- Describe the problem of fatigue in aviation with specific reference to work hours, duty periods, circadian disruption and insufficient sleep
- Explain the impact sleep deprivation can have on a pilot
- Discuss the Federal Aviation Administration crew rest regulations as defined by the Code of Federal Regulations
- Describe some of the key preflight, inflight and postflight countermeasures to fatigue
- Give examples of the use of hypnotics for improving sleep and alertness
- Give examples of wake promoters and sleep-inducing agents and describe the advantages and disadvantages of each
- Describe the relevant regulation and policies governing crew rest and duty limitations in military aviation.

2.1 Introduction

» A physiological state of reduced mental or physical performance capability resulting from sleep loss or extended wakefulness, circadian phase, or workload that can impair a crewmember's alertness and ability to safely operate an aircraft or perform safety-related duties.

- International Civil Aviation Organization definition of pilot fatigue

- March 19, 2016. FlyDubai Flight 981 crashes at Rostov-on-Don airport, killing 62 on board. The captain, Aristos Sokratous, had already resigned from the airline, citing exhaustion. He was serving out his three-month notice at the time of the accident. Following the accident, anonymous pilots employed by FlyDubai and Emirates who were interviewed by the press explained they were "dangerously tired".
- July 23, 2014. TransAsia Flight GE 222 crashes near Magong Airport, killing 47. Pilot fatigue is cited as a contributing factor.
- In October 2013, the British Civil Aviation Authority hit the headlines when it was revealed that a Virgin Atlantic Airbus 330 had operated on autopilot while both pilots slept after having only slept 5 hours in the previous 2 days. "Bad scheduling" was to blame.

Pilot fatigue is a serious problem in aviation operations. Changing work hours, time zone transitions and long duty periods combined with lack of sleep all conspire to cause fatigue. And the deleterious effects of that fatigue can have a pronounced impact on flight performance [1]. Put simply, pilots who are excessively fatigued make more mistakes than well-rested pilots. In the long term, chronically fatigued pilots are at higher risk for cardiovascular problems, gastrointestinal problems and weight gain than more rested pilots.

Ways to mitigate pilot fatigue stretch back to the 1930s, which is when flight time limitations and pilot sleep recommendations were introduced. Surprisingly, there have been no significant changes to aircrew scheduling since that time. This is surprising

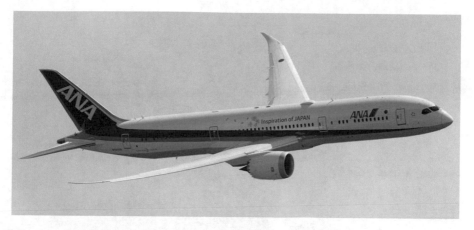

because of the wealth of available research on the subject of sleep and fatigue. That research reveals that each subset of pilots attribute their fatigue to a different set of circumstances. For example, long-haul pilots become fatigued as a result of constantly changing time zones and the sleep deprivation that is a consequence of constantly disrupted circadian rhythms. Domestic pilots on the other hand attribute their fatigue to high workload, multiple flight legs and sleep deprivation. Corporate pilots blame their fatigue on scheduling issues, late arrivals and early awakenings. Military pilots also suffer from excessive fatigue as a result of sleep restrictions, consecutive duty days, minimal rest periods and around-the-clock task demands. There is no end in sight for resolving the fatigue problem. In fact, if anything, the problem will become even more of a challenge with the advent of ultra-long range (ULR) aircraft (◘ Fig. 2.1) that fly 18, 19 or even 20 plus hours at a stretch.

2.2 Fatigue Physiology

So what exactly is fatigue? From a physiological perspective, research conducted inflight and in simulators has observed a number of characteristics. One of these characteristics is the effect of fatigue on alertness. There are three distinct factors that determine cockpit alertness: circadian rhythms, sleep pressure and sleep inertia. We'll begin with *circadian rhythms*.

2.2.1 Circadian Rhythms

Circadian rhythms comprise the biological and psychological processes that govern our internal clock. For example, body temperature, light, meals, work activity and alertness are processes that vary over the 24-hour day and which collectively are known as "circadian rhythms". The problem with these circadian rhythms is that it is difficult to adjust to new cyclical patterns of the processes that govern the rhythms [2]. This is

2

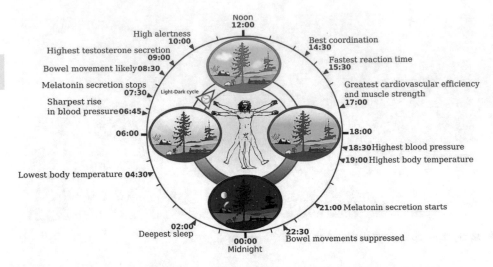

○ **Fig. 2.2** Overview of circadian rhythms. Our biological clock affects the daily rhythm of many physiological processes. This diagram depicts the circadian rhythms of someone who rises early in morning, eats lunch around noon, and sleeps at night. Although circadian rhythms tend to be synchronized with cycles of light and dark, other factors - such as ambient temperature, meal times, stress and exercise - can influence the timing. Credit: Inkscape by YassineMrabet

because we are hardwired to be asleep, to eat and to work at certain times of the day. Upset these timings, and people become discombobulated. Consider jet lag, which has a major disruptive effect on circadian rhythms. And when circadian rhythms are disrupted, alertness is compromised and fatigue is increased (○ Fig. 2.2).

For example, when flying eastbound, the day is shortened and the body must "advance" to a new rhythm, which means the first sleep is short, followed by a longer rest period. This process is known as *phase advance*. When traveling westbound, the day is lengthened and the first sleep is longer, followed by a shorter sleep period in a process known as *phase delay*. Making the whole adjustment more complicated is the *resynchronization of the circadian rhythms* (remember all those processes that comprise circadian rhythms?—they must *all* be reset). It is complicated because this process is asymmetrical. For westbound flights crossing eight or more time zones, it will take about 5 days for a 95% adjustment, whereas for eastbound flights that cross eight or more time zones, it takes 6.5 days to achieve 95% adjustment [2].

The next factor is sleep propensity or *sleep pressure*, which is simply the physiological need to sleep. When flying across multiple time zones, the accrued fatigue makes you want to nap, but while this strategy will improve wakefulness, it will not reset sleep propensity. Take a look at the graph again in ○ Fig. 2.2. Now imagine you're flying from Orlando to Kona, Hawaii. Kona is displaced by six time zones. So, if you take the early United Airlines flight out of Orlando at 0600 and arrive in Kona at around noon, you will have been awake for 12 hours already. But by the time 2100 rolls around, you will have been awake for 21 hours and your greatest need for sleep will have been at around 3:00 pm local time. This is when you will feel the most fatigued. So how does this fatigue manifest itself in terms of pilot performance? Take a look at ○ Table 2.1.

⬛ Table 2.1   Performance decrement after 16 and 24 hours

Variable	Baseline performance	Decrement after 16 h	Decrement after 24 h
Visual vigilance response time (sec)	0.43	×1.06	×1.15
Visual vigilance (% missed)	16%	×2.57	×4.56
Continuous memory recall response time (sec)	0.46	×1.16	×1.41
Continuous memory recall (% missed)	5%	×1.76	×3.10
Unstable tracking (RMS error)	329	×1.56	×2.49

2.2.1.1 Jet Lag and Phase Lag

Technically, jet lag occurs when the biological clock's processes are displaced by at least 3 hours. So, if you jump on a flight in Orlando and fly to Vancouver, you will experience a three-hour time difference, which means resetting your normal activities. For some people—pilots specifically—the problem of jet lag is compounded by *shift lag*, which means having to work when most people are sleeping and trying to sleep when most people are working. Imagine you're a pilot flying the 0200 Spirit Airlines flight from San Jose, Costa Rica, to Fort Lauderdale, Florida, and you have to catch some shuteye mid-morning. This is shift lag. Like jet lag, shift lag poses similar short-term problems related to fatigue. Generally, adjusting to a new time zone (jet lag) is easier than adjusting to a new nonstandard sleep/wake cycle [2].

2.2.1.2 Combating Jet Lag

What can pilots and passengers do to reduce the effect of jet lag and reset their circadian rhythms? Melatonin, a hormone produced in the brain, has been shown to synchronize circadian mechanisms in the cells. When administered as a drug (the usual dose is anywhere between 0.5 mg and 5 mg), it can advance the body's clock between 1300 and 0100 with a peak response at 1600. In some countries, melatonin is licensed to treat insomnia. Yet melatonin [3] has mixed reviews, so what else can pilots and passengers do? Altering meal times is another strategy, since food is a strong timing cue for the body. Adjusting your meal times to another destination's clock is pretty simple, although you might feel hungry for while. Unfortunately, despite hundreds of controlled studies investigating circadian rhythms and jet lag, the usual cliché applies: more research needs to be conducted to evaluate ways of reprogramming circadian rhythms.

2.2.1.3 Research

We know that jet lag and shift lag conspire to produce fatigue, but what sort of metrics can be used to measure just how tired a pilot might be? One feature of fatigue common to all pilots is impairment of central nervous system functioning. For example, long-haul pilots are prone to lapses in attention and vigilance during periods of low workload. Research [4] that documented these lapses used electroencephalography (EEG) to measure periods of slow-wave EEG activity in pilots during the fourth and fifth hour of flight. The results showed that the EEG activity was very similar to that exhibited by those about to fall asleep.

Similar research studies [5, 6] revealed that micro-sleeps occurred nine times more often during nighttime flights than daytime flights, and—worryingly!—that these micro-sleeps were not usually noticed by the flight crew. And these micro-sleeps also occurred during the final 90 minutes of flight, with some pilots nodding off up to six times for up to 5 seconds during the landing phase! Surveys back up these research findings, as evidenced by a NASA survey of fatigue among pilots. In this survey, 80% of pilots (1,424 flight crewmembers) reported having fallen asleep during a flight. The bottom line: 7% *of all civil aviation accidents may be attributed to fatigue.* And in the military, that statistic is even more sobering: between 1974 and 1990, one quarter of the USAF's night tactical fighter accidents were the result of fatigue. The problem is that humans are not designed to deal with multiple time zone changes, excessive sleep deprivation, nonstandard shift patterns or around-the-clock missions. This is why it is necessary to manage fatigue, and one way to do this is through regulations.

2.3 Current Regulations

2.3.1 FAA Regulations

The FAA regulates crew rest for civilian aviation in the Code of Federal Regulations (CFRs) sub-part 91.1057 (Aside). In addition to defining crew rest, these regulations also define minimum mandatory rest periods which is 10 hours before a duty period (Aside). This may sound like a reasonable amount of time, and in most cases it is, but this time period includes local travel time to and from the place of rest. Obviously, including the local travel time within the definition of rest time reduces the actual amount of rest time a crew has. It is for this reason that many flight crews are unable to log 8 hours of uninterrupted sleep. For example, if a crew lands at Kona, Hawaii, and is staying at the Royal Kona Resort in downtown Kona, they are faced with a 30-minute drive to and from the airport on a good day. And that time doesn't include transiting through the airport or registering at the hotel. Then there is the subject of personal needs to take care of, such as eating.

Aside

§ 91.1057 Flight, Duty and Rest Time Requirements: All Crewmembers.

Rest period means a period of time required pursuant to this subpart that is free of all responsibility for work or duty prior to the commencement of, or following completion of, a duty period, and during which the flight crewmember or flight attendant cannot be required to receive contact from the program manager. A rest period does not include any time during which the program manager imposes on a flight crewmember or flight attendant any duty or restraint, including any actual work or present responsibility for work should the occasion arise.

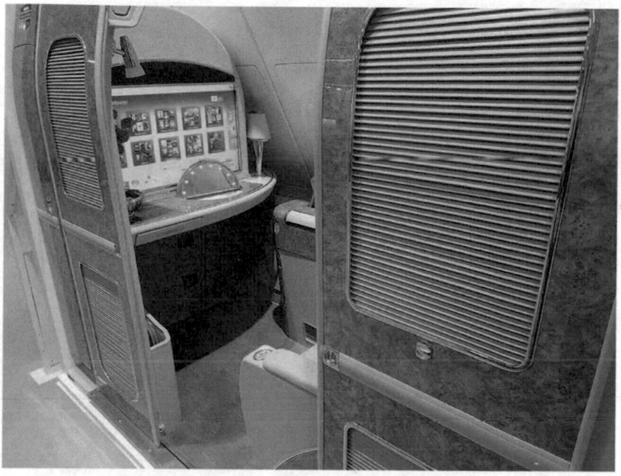

◘ Fig. 2.3 Airbus A380 first class private suite. Credit: Travelarz

For augmented crews, duty time regulations are slightly different. An *augmented crew* is one composed of more than the minimum number required to operate the aircraft. For this crew category, the rest period is 12 hours and is increased to 18 hours for flights that cross several time zones. It sounds like an improvement, but it should be highlighted that the extended time period does not include time set aside for the timing of sleep as it corresponds with circadian phases. Take the Emirates (◘ Fig. 2.3) flight from Orlando to Dubai as an example. This flight, which takes 13 hours and 50 minutes, is one of the longest flights in the world. It departs Orlando at 1330 local time and arrives in Dubai at 1220 local time. With a time zone differential of 8 hours, pilots arriving in Dubai do so with their body clocks set at 0420 Orlando time. Try going to sleep for 10 hours starting at 5 in the morning![1]

Before examining the ways fatigue can be mitigated, we need to remind ourselves what the industry definitions of duty time and flight time are. As you can see in the CFR definition (Aside), *duty period* includes flight time, which begins when the aircraft moves from its parked position at its departure airport and ends when it comes to a stop at its destination airport. Basically, flight time is a component of duty time and generally duty time is longer than flight time because it includes the time between when aircrew report for a flight and when they are released from that flight. As you can see in ◘ Tables 2.2a and 2.2b the maximum allowable flight time and the maximum allowable duty time are different for different crews. One key difference between these crew categories is that augmented crews cannot work longer than 8 hours on the flight deck. Augmented crews also have access to rest facilities (◘ Fig. 2.4).

1 A discussion of even some of the research that has been conducted on the subject of fatigue is beyond the scope of this publication. If you are interested in a detailed assessment, I refer you to John Caldwell's book *Fatigue in Aviation: A Guide to Staying Awake at the Stick* published by Routledge.

2

§ 91.1057 Flight, Duty and Rest Time Requirements: All Crewmembers.

Duty period means the period of elapsed time between reporting for an assignment involving flight time and release from that assignment by the program manager. All time between these two points is part of the duty period, even if flight time is interrupted by non-flight-related duties. The time is calculated using either Coordinated Universal Time or local time to reflect the total elapsed time.

▢ Table 2.2a   Minimum rest periods and maximum flight and duty periods for non-augmented and augmented crews

	Non-augmented crew (single or two-pilot crew)	Augmented crew
Minimum pre-duty rest period	10 h	10 h
Minimum post-duty rest period	10 h	12 h 18 h for multiple time zones
Maximum flight time	10 h	12 h
Maximum duty time	14 h	16 h
Maximum duty time 1 week	30 h	30 h
Maximum duty time 1 month	100 h	100 h
Maximum duty time 1 year	1400 h	1400 h

2.3.2 Military Regulations

While the details of military mishaps are not as freely available as NTSB reports, fatigue is just as much of a concern for the military as it is for civil aviation. In fact, the US Navy and the Marine Corps have identified fatigue as the primary cause of Class A accidents (mishaps that exceed one million dollars and include a fatality or a destroyed aircraft) between 1990 and 2011. In many instances, military pilots have higher demands placed upon them than civilian pilots because in addition to the shift lag, military aviators often have to fly in wartime operations. Compounding that stress is the added challenge of pressure—military pilots often have no choice whether or not to make a flight due to the repercussions if they decide not to fly. Because of these factors, it is perhaps not surprising that the fatigue management policies implemented by the military (Aside) are not nearly as complex as the civil aviation regulations: Army Regulation 385–95, 10 January 2000; Air Force Instruction 11-202 v3, 5 April 2006; OPNAV Instruction 3710.7T, 1 March 2004.

Table 2.2b Maximum flight duty period hours

Aircraft type	Basic aircrew	Augmented aircrew
Single piloted aircraft	12	NA
Fighter attack or trainer (dual control)	12	16
Bomber, reconnaissance. Electronic warfare or battle management (dual control)	16	24
Tanker/transport	16	NA
Tanker/transport with sleeping provisions	16	24
Rotary wing (without auto flight control systems)	12	14
Rotary wing (with auto flight control systems)	14	18
Utility	12	18
Unmanned aircraft system (single control)	12	NA
Unmanned aircraft system (dual control)	16	NA
Tilt-rotor	16	NA

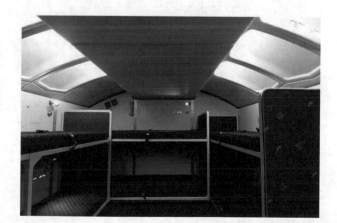

Fig. 2.4 A multiple-bunk class 1 crew rest compartment. The Federal Aviation Administration defines three classes of crew rest facilities, dependent on the number of crew and the duration of the flight. Crew rest periods may be provided in higher classed rest areas than required; for example, some airplanes may not have a class 2 rest facility, providing breaks in a crew rest. Rest facility classifications from highest to lowest: **Class 1 rest facility:** This class requires access to an area physically separated from the flight deck and the passenger cabin; bunks or other flat areas for sleeping; provisions for sound and lighting isolation. **Class 2 rest facility:** This class requires access to at least a lie-flat seat and separation from passengers by a curtain. **Class 3 rest facility:** This class only requires a cabin seat that is able to recline and has foot support. Credit: A. Katranzhi

2

Aside

Military (USAF) Flight Duty Period[2]

2.1. Crew Rest. Crew rest is compulsory for aircrewmembers prior to performing any duties involving aircraft operations and is a minimum of 12 non-duty hours before the Flight Duty Period (FDP) begins (T-2). Crew rest is free time and includes time for meals, transportation, and rest. This time must include an opportunity for at least 8 hours of uninterrupted sleep. Crew rest period cannot begin until after the completion of official duties.

2.1.1. Aircrewmembers are individually responsible to ensure they obtain sufficient rest during a crew rest period. 2.1.2. Once crew rest begins, any official business interrupts the crew rest period. If crew rest is interrupted, individuals will immediately inform appropriate leadership or command and control (C2) and will either begin a new crew rest period or not perform flight duties (T-2). Exception: PIC (or designee) may initiate mission-related communication with official agencies without interrupting crew rest.

2.1.3. Exceptions to the 12-Hour Minimum Crew Rest Periods. For continuous operations when basic aircrew FDPs are between 12 to 14 hours, subsequent crew rest may be reduced to a minimum of 10 hours by the PIC in order to maintain a 24-hour work/rest schedule (T-2). "Continuous operations" is defined as three or more consecutive FDPs of at least 12 hours duration with minimum crew rest period. 2.1.3.1. The 10-hour crew rest exception shall only be used to keep crews in 24-hour clock cycles, not for scheduling convenience or additional sortie generation (T-2). 2.1.3.2. Any reduction from 12-hour crew rest requires pre-coordination for transportation, meals, and quarters so that crewmembers are provided an opportunity for at least 8 hours of uninterrupted sleep (T-2).

US Air Force Guidance for Scheduling Flight Missions to Avoid Fatigue in Aircrew[3]

- Provisions should be made for augmenting flight crews when possible to permit inflight rest periods.

- Cockpit naps (taken by one crewmember at a time) of up to 45 min in duration are authorized during noncritical flight phases. Multiple naps permitted when feasible.
- Crew bunks or other suitable rest facilities should be provided on board aircraft when possible.
- Adequate crew rest is required prior to flight duty periods. Normally, this means 12 h off duty every 24 h. There should be a minimum of 10 h of restful time that includes an opportunity for at least 8 h of uninterrupted sleep during the 12 h preceding the flight duty period.
- Shorter off-duty periods of 10 h may be used as an exception in continuous operations, but this exception should be minimized, and after several days of shorter off-duty periods, commanders should provide sufficient rest to counter cumulative fatigue.
- Maximum flying time should be limited to 56 h per 7 d, 125 h per 30 d, and 330 h per 90 consecutive days.
- If non-flight duties significantly extend the overall duty period (by 2 h or more), consideration should be given to reducing the number of allowed flight hours.
- Generally speaking, the maximum flight duty period for any given day should fall within the range of 12 to16 h in situations where crew augmentation is not possible.
- When augmented crews are an option, duty days normally can extend to 16–24 h (in the case of the B-2 Bomber, some missions extend to 44 h).
- Factors affecting maximum flight duty period include: single vs. multi-seat aircraft, level of automation, availability of onboard rest facilities, and type of flight mission.
- Alertness management strategies such as techniques to promote pre-duty sleep, extended crew rest periods, controlled cockpit rest, bright light exposure, activity breaks, pharmacological sleep and alertness aids, and fatigue management education should be implemented as appropriate.

---

2   AFI11-202V3_AFGM2017-01 2 OCTOBER 2017 MEMORANDUM FOR DISTRIBUTION C MAJCOMs/ FOAs/DRUs FROM: HQ USAF/A3 1480.

3   AFI 11-202 Volume 3, General Flight Rules.

2.4 Countermeasures

2.4.1 Fatigue Risk Management (FRMS)

>> A data-driven means of continuously monitoring and managing fatigue-related safety risks, based on scientific principles and knowledge as well as operational experience that aims to ensure relevant personnel are performing at adequate levels of alertness.

   - ICAO definition of FRMS, 2011

One regulatory countermeasures approach is the FRMS (◘ Fig. 2.5). This system addresses the physiological and operational aspects of fatigue. It is based on scientific research [7] and it has gained the attention of a number of aviation regulatory groups around the world. Some of these groups, such as the US-based Flight Safety Foundation and the Civil Aviation Authority in Australia, recommend requirements for an effective FRMS. For example, the Flight Safety Foundation [7] suggests the following guidelines be implemented as part of an effective FRMS:

- Develop a fatigue risk management policy
- Formalize education/awareness training programs
- Create a crew fatigue-reporting mechanism with associated feedback, procedures, and measures for monitoring fatigue levels
- Develop procedures for reporting, investigating, and recording incidents in which fatigue was a factor
- Implement processes and procedures for evaluating information on fatigue levels and fatigue-related incidents, implementing interventions, and evaluating their effects.

◘ **Fig. 2.5** FRMS. Credit: IATA

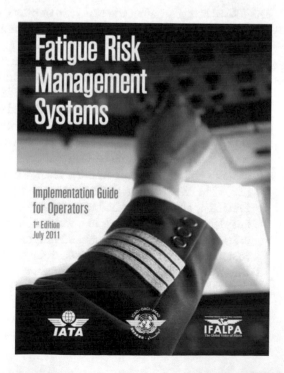

The Civil Aviation Safety Authority (Australian Government Civil Aviation Authority) on the other hand, suggests a FRMS should consider:
- Sleep opportunity provided by schedules
- Sleep obtained by personnel to indicate fitness for duty
- Hours of wakefulness
- Circadian factors
- Sleep disorders
- Operational demographics

All these recommendations make for encouraging reading, but what about implementation? Guidelines are in place in the form of the Fatigue Management Guide for Airline Operations, which was developed by the ICAO and the International Federation of Airline Pilots (IFALPA). This publication also supports FRMS (Appendix II) and it provides operators with a comprehensive set of prescriptive and performance-base management approaches. The 167-page guide is available as a free download via FRMS@ iata.org. As far as widespread regulation is concerned, FRMS has a way to go, but there are examples of successful systems in place:
- **New Zealand** has accrued a long experience of applying FRMS principles. In 1995 the New Zealand Civil Aviation Authority allowed operators to implement FRMS, and in 2014 it established the Fatigue Risk Management Panel (FRMP) that:

> » Facilitates the development of the aviation community expert views on fatigue management, and provides advice and information to the CAA on those issues. It will facilitate the development of documentation and associated resources, and monitor progress on these issues.[4]

The FRMP brings together the expertise of pilots, engineers, cabin crew and air traffic controllers and provides a forum for the exchange of information related to fatigue-related risks in the country's aviation system.
- **Singapore**. Singapore Airlines (SIA). This carrier adopted FRMS in 2003 following the introduction its ultra-long haul flight (ULF) from Singapore to New York. Then, in 2014, the Civil Aviation Authority of Singapore (CAAS) introduced new fatigue management regulations that included a requirement that pilots not fly more than two night flights per week. In addition to the night restriction, SIA also changed its flight crew roster on some of its ULFs. For example, its Tokyo to Los Angeles flight crew was increased from one captain and two first officers to two captains and a first officer. Another change it made to this flight was requiring only two of the crew to be on the flight deck at any one time while the third rested. Previously all three crew had to be present on the flight deck.
- **EasyJet**. EasyJet is a European low-cost, short-haul carrier that implemented a crew roster pattern that considered fatigue management principles. The original roster comprised three early starts, three late starts and three days, off whereas the amended roster comprised a sequence of five early starts followed by two days off and five late starts. EasyJet has since implemented a Human Factors

Monitoring Program (HFMP) to develop the methodology of fatigue management in partnership with NASA Ames and Imperial College in London. The airline also conducts a biennial analysis of crew rosters that includes assessments of objective and subjective methodologies, with the aim of identifying fatigue precursors.

2.4.2 Sleep-Promoting Substances

What happens if you happen to be an airline pilot who, even after adopting the most effective sleep scheduling, exercise *and* nutrition strategies, still has trouble falling asleep? That is where it may be necessary to examine medical alertness-enhancing options. The good news is there are myriad products available that will keep you awake. The bad news is that most of these products should not be adopted as the default replacement for rest and/or sleep. Many of these products have side effects, and some may cause long-term issues with sleep architecture.

One of the most popular non-FDA-regulated medicines used to assist in falling asleep is melatonin (see earlier discussion on jet lag). When taken to alleviate insomnia during regular nighttime hours, it has been proven to be very effective [3]. But when taken outside regular nighttime hours, as would be the case when traveling across time zones to advance the sleep period for instance, melatonin may exert mild hypnotic effects. The problem is that the effectiveness of melatonin is to some extent determined by the extent of the circadian phase delay and also by the state of circadian desynchrony that may already exist. For example, a pilot who has made multiple trips across multiple time zones in two weeks will be suffering from more circadian desynchrony than a pilot who has made just one long haul flight in that same period. The problem is that most pilots—and most scientists, to be fair—do not have a detailed understanding about the efficacy of melatonin when applied to circadian shifts.

Another non-FDA-regulated substance is valerian [8]. While this herb (the product Sleep MD™ is valerian-based) has not been clinically proven to treat insomnia, it has been shown to be very effective in promoting sleep.

2.4.2.1 Caffeine

To promote alertness, coffee is by far the most popular non-FDA-regulated fatigue countermeasure (although Red Bull seems to be catching up!) thanks to its magic ingredient: caffeine (◘ Fig. 2.6). Study after study *after study* has shown just how effective caffeine is in improving vigilance in those who have been deprived of sleep. Not only is caffeine (in moderation) safe and effective, but its effects also start almost immediately and last for 5 or 6 hours. But not all caffeine (◘ Table 2.3) is the same, and not all people react to it the same way. For one thing, regular caffeine use leads to tolerance. This means that your daily Starbucks may not give you as much of a caffeine-kick a year from now. Most people understand this, which is why some seek out drinks containing more caffeine. The problem with this strategy is that if you drink too much caffeine, you may begin to suffer side effects such as rapid heart rate, insomnia, dehydration, nervousness and irritable bowel syndrome. The key? Tactical caffeine use—basically, use caffeine only when you really need it.

2

» Without proper management, ultra-long-range operations may exacerbate the fatigue levels that have already been shown to impair safety, alertness and performance in existing flight operations.

- Quote from position paper on the subject of pilot fatigue published by the Aerospace Medical Association in 2009.

◘ **Fig. 2.6**   Coffee. Most pilots can't fly without this! Credit: Julius Schorzman

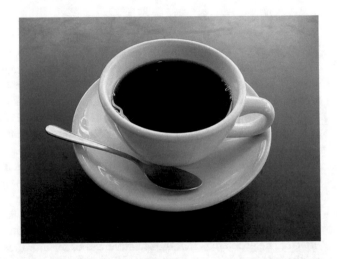

◘ **Table 2.3**   Over-the-counter caffeine drinks

Drink	Caffeine content
Starbucks® Tall	250 mg
Starbucks® Grande	375 mg
Coke®	50 mg
Black tea[a]	50 mg
2 Excedrin®	130 mg
Red Bull®	80 mg
Black Insomnia Coffee	702 mg
Dunkin Donuts Iced Coffee (24 fl oz)	297 mg
Jolt Endurance Shot (2 fl oz)	200 mg
McDonalds Coffee (16 fl oz)	145 mg
Mountain Dew (12 fl oz)	54 mg

[a]There are large variations in the strength of black tea. For example, Earl Grey has a lower caffeine content than Darjeeling, which in turn has a lower caffeine content than Orange Pekoe

2.5 Ultra-Long-Range Flights

As technology advances and aircraft such as the Airbus A350-900ULR become lighter and more fuel efficient, flights have become longer, and longer, and *longer*. With the advent of Airbus's Ultra Long Range A350, which will have a range of 17,960 km, it won't be long before passengers will be able to fly direct from Sydney to London. Such mind-numbingly long flights are known as ultra-long-haul flights and are defined as any flight that takes 16 hours or more. These flights are a relatively new phenomenon, having been around since 2004 when Singapore Airlines started flying from Singapore to Newark, a 19-hour flight that covered 15,300 km. The route was discontinued in 2013 when rising fuel prices made the flight uneconomical. Since fuel prices recovered in 2014, there has been a trend among the airlines to advertise longer and longer routes. But are the pilots on these flights getting enough rest? (◘ Table 2.4)

To answer this question, let's turn to research. For the purposes of this chapter, we'll discuss a report published in the December 2014 issue of *Aviation, Space and Environmental Medicine*, which examined the effectiveness of fatigue mitigation measures applied to pilots flying ULR flights [9]. This paper studied 52 pilots flying a westbound ULR from Johannesburg, South Africa, to Kennedy International, New York. During their flights, the pilots wore an actigraph (◘ Fig. 2.7) that monitored rest and activity cycles before, during and after their flights.

◘ Table 2.4   Evolution of ultra-long flights

Airline	City Pair	Aircraft	Distance	Flight hours	Year of operation	Hub
Singapore Airlines	Singapore and New York	A340-500	15,343 km	18.5 h	2004–2013	Singapore
Qantas	Sydney and Dallas	A380	13,815 km	15 h 30 m	2014	Sydney
Emirates	Dubai and Panama City	B777	13,825 km	17 h 35 m	2015	Dubai
Emirates	Dubai and Auckland	B777	14,200 km	17 h 15 m	2016	Dubai
Qatar Airways	Doha and Auckland	B777	14,529 km	17 h 30 m	2017	Doha
Singapore Airlines	Singapore and New York	A350-900ULR	16,500 km	19 h	2018	Singapore
United Airlines	Houston and Sydney	B787-9	14,000 km	17 h 55 m	2018	Houston
Qantas	Perth – London	B787	14,466 km	17 h	2018	Sydney
Qantas	Sydney – London	?	16,983 km	20 h 20 m	2022	Sydney

2

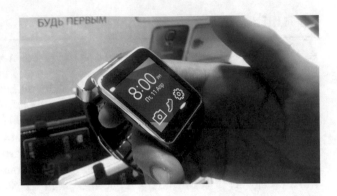

Three days before their flights, the four pilots, two of whom were designated as primary crew and two of whom were support crew, were given their suggested preflight and inflight rest schedule. The outbound flight was divided into four (3, 4, 4 and 3 hours) rest breaks and each pilot received two breaks. To reduce wakefulness before the approach and landing phase, the primary crew was advised to take the second and fourth rest breaks. The flights were flown in an Airbus A340-600s that departed Johannesburg at 2100 local time, arriving at Kennedy 17 hours later, at 1400 Johannesburg time (0700 Kennedy time). After a 48-hour layover, the return flight departed Kennedy at 1030 local time (1730 Johannesburg time), arriving 14 hours and 30 minutes later at 0100 Kennedy time (0800 Johannesburg time). After each preflight, inflight and postflight sleep period, the pilots rated their sleep quality from 1 (extremely good) to 7 (extremely poor). They also rated their fatigue level before and after each sleep period from 1 (fully alert) to 7 (completely exhausted) and their sleepiness from 1 (extremely alert) to 9 (extremely sleepy). Their performance was assessed using a vigilance task that required the pilots to look at a display on a screen and push a button when a symbol appeared [9].

During their layovers, the pilots slept an average of 33 minutes longer in the first 24 hours than during their normal sleep period, whereas during the final 24 hours the pilots averaged 35 minutes less sleep. All the pilots had their longest sleeps during New York night. Following the ULR flight, pilots logged one hour more sleep during the first 24 hours compared with their normal sleep pattern. Two days after completing their trips, sleep duration across all pilots returned to nominal levels, although pilots reported feeling more fatigued on waking on the first day postflight.

On the outbound and inbound legs, the pilots took advantage of at least two inflight rest breaks and 70% of the crew tried to take their rest breaks in the rest facilities. On the outbound leg, the sleep duration and quality was about the same as for the primary and secondary crew, but on the inbound leg the secondary crew reported less sleep than the primary crew.

So what did the researchers find? Data analysis suggested *a pattern of gradually increasing fatigue across the flight, with slight decreases in fatigue following each inflight sleep period*. The PVT data also revealed *a general pattern of slower performance across the flight, with the exception of primary crew on the outbound flight*. Generally, the report concluded that the suggested rest-break pattern had been effective in reducing crew fatigue and sleepiness during the final flight phases. The researchers also agreed that a westbound ULR flight can be safely managed using a range of mitigation strategies, and that resulting fatigue levels are no worse, and in fact in many instances are better, than the return non-ULR flight. For the pilots, these mitigation strategies included an augmented crew and advice about which rest strategies to adopt. One piece of advice the study pilots did not follow was to stay on domicile time during their layover. Instead, the pilots waited until nighttime New York time before starting their sleep period. The pilots' reason for this was attributed to social engagements and local attractions, which prompted the researchers to amend their advice to recommending that pilots increase their sleep time before the return flight. In terms of recovery, it was noted that almost complete recovery was reported by the pilots 4 days after returning to Johannesburg.

In 2018, the FAA began applying a case-by-case approach to approving ULR pairs. This approval is done by the FAA issuing a nonstandard operations specification paragraph known as Operations Specification (OpSpec) A332, which is issued by the Air Transportation Division (AFS-200). If an airline is interested in implementing a new ULR flight, it applies to the FAA and the FAA reviews the route. It conducts this review by consulting the operational implications, duty times, flight times, rest periods, and the scientific literature. To assist those in the FAA conducting this assessment, the FAA has adopted the Sleep, Activity, Fatigue and task Effectiveness (SAFTE)™ fatigued model[5] invented by IBR (Institutes for Behavioral Resources, Inc.) President Dr. Steven Hursh.

Another model used by the FAA is the Fatigue Avoidance Scheduling Tool (FAST), which is also used by the Department of Transportation and the Department of Defense to assess fatigue. Over the years, the SAFTE/FAST combination has proven an accurate and reliable means by which to identify fatigue risk factors, which is why it is applied to ULR city pair proposals. Having said that, an air carrier is not limited to using the SAFTE/FAST when applying for its OpSec A332 approval.

2.6 Sleep and Sleep Deprivation

Most people need about seven to eight hours of sleep in each 24-hour period. Some need more and some need less. Unfortunately, although many of us do our best to fit in those seven or eight hours, many of us are still sleep-deprived. And some of those who are sleep-deprived may be losing sleep due to a sleep disorder. We'll get to the subject of sleep disorders soon, but first we need to understand the nature of sleep.

2.6.1 What is Sleep?

The "golden age" of sleep research was kick-started by Dr. Nathaniel Kleitman, a Professor Emeritus in Physiology at the University of Chicago, where he was known as the "father of sleep research". It was Kleitman who proposed the existence of a

---

5   SAFTE is a patented computerized model that predicts changes in cognitive performance based on a person's sleep/wake cycle.

rest-activity cycle and co-discovered (together with Eugene Aserinsky) REM sleep. Many of Kleitman's research subjects were family and friends, but the professor also experimented on himself, once staying awake for 180 hours straight to study the effects of sleep deprivation. Until Kleitman's work in the late 1950s, most people thought of sleep as a dormant and passive part of our lives. Now, thanks to Kleitman, we know that our brains are very active during sleep. The chemicals that control whether we are asleep or awake arc known as *neurotransmitters*. Groups of neurons in our brains produce neurotransmitters such as serotonin that either "switch on" to keep us awake or "switch off" to send us to sleep. While we are asleep, we pass through five distinct phases (also known as *ultradian rhythms*), the first four of which are characterized as non-REM sleep and the fifth which is known as REM sleep [10, 11]. You can see how much time you typically spend in each cycle in the hypnogram depicted in ◘ Fig. 2.8.

The first cycle is usually about 90 minutes, and each successive cycle is typically about 100 to 120 minutes. Some individuals have longer and some have shorter cycles, but generally each cycle follows the stages of non-REM sleep stages 1 through 4 before entering REM sleep. In Stage 1 we experience light sleep and can be woken easily, whereas Stage 2 is slightly deeper sleep that is characterized by eye movements and

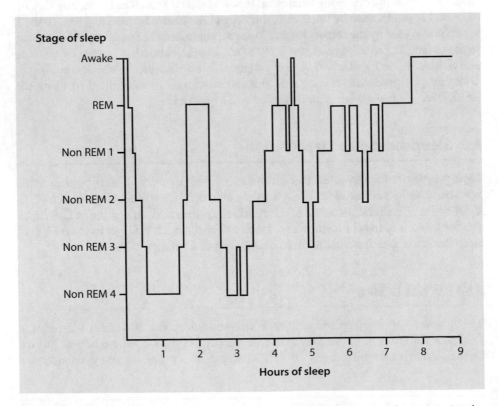

◘ Fig. 2.8   Example of a hypnogram of a normal, healthy adult. This hypnogram shows stage 3 and stage 4. Credit: Tash510

fluctuations in the electrical activity of the brain. By the time we enter Stages 3 and 4, our brain activity is a mix of slow waves known as delta waves and smaller, faster waves. This is deep sleep, and there is no eye movement or muscle activity. If you happen to be woken from this sleep stage you will feel very groggy and extremely discombobulated. Finally, we enter REM sleep and our breathing becomes irregular and more rapid. Our heart rate increases and our blood pressure rise. Another characteristic of this stage is vivid dreams.

2.6.2 Quality of Sleep

Those neurotransmitters mentioned earlier are influenced in all sorts of ways, and it is the way they are influenced that determines sleep and wakefulness. For example, what we eat and what medication we take can trigger different neurotransmitter signals that in turn make us feel alert or drowsy. Take caffeine, for instance. Even in moderation, caffeine intake produces wakefulness and alertness, but an excessive intake can result in insomnia and altered sleep architecture. Alcohol is another sleep-altering substance. Some people drink alcohol to help them fall asleep, but this strategy robs people of their REM sleep, which means the sleep they get is not restorative. Other people are especially sensitive to temperature, which in turn can disrupt REM sleep. Some guidelines: don't drink before going to sleep, be sure to drink your final caffeine-containing beverage of the day at least 6 hours before you go to sleep, choose a comfortable mattress, and sleep in a quiet bedroom.

2.6.3 Sleep Debt and Sleep Deprivation

So, how much sleep do we really need? If you happen to be a teenager, then you need about nine hours a night. Adults can make do with seven or eight, but these are average numbers. Some people function just fine on four hours (!) of sleep, while others need their daily ten hours of shuteye every night. No matter how much sleep you need, the bottom line is that if you don't get enough, you will enter into a state of *sleep debt*, and this is not something anyone can adapt to. Sleep debt is a little like being overdrawn at the bank—eventually you have to pay back that debt. If you don't, then you enter into a state of *sleep deprivation*. Sleep deprivation is dangerous (◘ Table 2.5). Studies on rats

◘ Table 2.5	Effects of sleep deprivation
After 24 hours	Deterioration in performance of tasks that are newly learned or that require vigilance
After 36 hours	A marked deterioration in ability to register and understand information
After 72 hours	Performance on most tasks will be about 50 percent of normal
3–4 days	This is the limit for intensive work. Visual illusions are likely at this stage.

have found that rats who are deprived of REM sleep live only five weeks, which is a dramatic reduction from their normal lifespan of two to three years. Deprive these rats of all sleep entirely, and their life expectancy drops to three weeks, which is a little longer than we humans perform: after 12 days without sleep, we may die.

2.6.4 Sleep Disorders

There are close to 100 medically recognized sleep disorders, classified into four categories:
1. Dysomnias. These describe disorders in which a person finds it difficult getting to sleep or maintaining sleep. One example is *sleep apnea syndrome*. Another example is *periodic limb movement in sleep* (PLMS).
2. Parasomnias. This category is characterized by problems that occur while sleeping.
3. Other sleep-disrupting disorders associated with psychiatric problems
4. Sleep-related disorders difficult to define.

A thorough discussion of these disorders is beyond the scope of this chapter, so we will limit ourselves to a brief review of some of those first-category disorders. We'll begin with sleep apnea, but before we continue, it is important to note that if a sleep disorder is suspected, a correct diagnosis is important, because without this, proper treatment cannot be prescribed. Those who think they have a sleep disorder should consult a sleep specialist, who may suggest an overnight stay in a sleep laboratory to determine the exact cause. Those who are interested in this topic may find the following websites of interest:

- **American Association of Sleep Medicine** ▶ www.aasm.org
- **National Sleep Foundation** ▶ www.sleepfoundation.org

2.6.4.1 Sleep Apnea

This disorder (◘ Fig. 2.9) is characterized by a cessation of breathing while sleeping for at least ten seconds. Sleep apnea is a normal occurrence while sleeping, as a normal person will experience up to four or five sleep apneas every hour and not suffer any effects the next day. But when this number climbs past 20, then daytime alertness suffers. Some people with severe sleep apnea may stop breathing as a many as *100 times every hour*, and some of these episodes may last more than a minute. Unfortunately, those with sleep apnea do not wake up every time an episode strikes, but they will usually complain of headaches, sleepiness, and depression the following day. Left untreated, sleep apnea can lead to serious health issues such as high blood pressure and stroke. Treatment includes continuous positive airway pressure (CPAP) and weight loss. CPAP (◘ Fig. 2.10) requires that the patient wear a small mask linked to an air pump that sends air through the mask and holds the airways open.

If a civil aviation pilot is diagnosed with sleep apnea, that pilot may still fly so long as treatment is ongoing and if that treatment is successful. One way of determining if that treatment has been successful is by completing the Maintenance of Wakefulness Test (MWT). If the pilot can pass the MWT, then he/she is deemed fit for duty.

Fig. 2.9 Airway obstruction during sleep. Credit: Drcamachoent

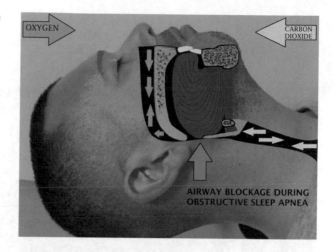

Fig. 2.10 CPAP machine with two models of full face masks. Credit: Zboralski

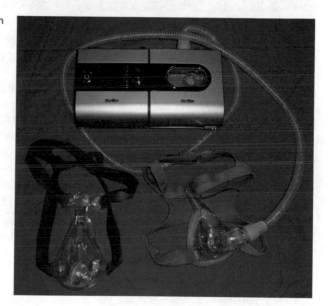

» It is defined as difficulty initiating or maintaining sleep, or non-restorative sleep for longer than one month resulting in impairment such as cognitive dysfunction and irritability.

- Definition of insomnia, *Army Aviation Magazine*

2.6.4.2 Insomnia

Insomnia, which affects between 10 to 15% of the US population, isn't technically regarded as a disorder, but rather a symptom or series of symptoms caused by lack of sleep and/or worry about sleep disruption. Those suffering from insomnia (■ Table 2.6) typically suffer a host of symptoms, including difficulty falling asleep, difficulty staying

Table 2.6 Types of insomnia

Types of insomnia	Duration	Causes
Transient insomnia	A few nights	Stress, noise, temperature changes, sleep/wake schedule (jet lag/shift work), medication side effects
Short-term insomnia	Two to four weeks of poor sleep	Stress, noise, temperature changes, sleep/wake schedule (jet lag/shift work), medication side effects
Chronic insomnia	Poor sleep most nights lasting a month or longer	Combination of factors related to transient and short-term insomnia. Common causes of chronic insomnia is depression. Other causes may include kidney disease, heart failure, asthma, sleep problems such as apnea, and behavioral factors such as caffeine or alcohol consumption

asleep, waking up too early, feeling physically and mentally drained during the day, nodding off during the day, feeling anxious and depressed at bedtime, and having trouble concentrating and remembering things [12].

Needless to say, suffering from insomnia is not conducive to a career in the aviation industry—or any industry for that matter. So what can you do if you happen to be an insomniac pilot who regularly nods off in the middle of a flight? You should try to regulate your sleep patterns as much as possible. This means avoiding caffeine intake close to your usual sleep time, limiting naps during the day, avoiding glances at the clock at night, and switching off you cellphone or keeping it out of eyesight. In fact, avoid any screen time—computer screen, video screens and *especially* that cellphone screen—before bed as much as possible. If all else fails, then consider Ambien, a pharmacologic sleep treatment that has been approved for pilots.

2.7 Summary

Now that you have read this chapter, you should understand that fatigue is a complex, multidimensional, non-specific and subjective complaint. It can cause cognitive and motor function compromise due to physiological and psychological impairments in performance, increased reaction times, reduced attention and reduced psychomotor performance. These can all conspire to reduce a pilot's ability to control an aircraft. Due to working shifts and the effects of jet lag, pilots are particularly susceptible to fatigue, which is why it is so important to employ the most effective countermeasures and treatments to combat the condition. Regulations and directives continue to be evaluated, especially with the recent advent of ULRs, but as we have seen in the Fly-Dubai incident, these regulations are not always implemented as rigorously as they should be.

Key Terms

CFRs - Code of Federal Regulations

CPAP - Continuous Positive Airway Pressure

FARs - Federal Aviation Regulations

FAST - Fatigue Avoidance Scheduling Tool

FDP - Flight Duty Period

FRMS - Fatigue Risk Management System

FSF - Flight Safety Foundation

HFMP - Human Factors Monitoring Program

MWT - Maintenance of Wakefulness Test

PLMS - Periodic Limb Movement in Sleep

PVT - Psychomotor Vigilance Test

SAFTE - Sleep, Activity and Fatigue Task Effectiveness

SIRA - System Integrated Risk Assessment

ULR - Ultra-long Range

Review Questions
1. Describe how fatigue can affect pilot performance
2. What is mean by the terms *phase delay* and *phase advance*?
3. Identify the maximum flight duty hours for basic aircrew
4. What are ultra-long flights?
5. Discuss the efficacy of current fatigue countermeasures
6. Briefly describe the FRMS approach to fatigue management
7. Distinguish between sleep debt and sleep deprivation
8. What is sleep apnea?
9. Describe some of the non-FDA regulated substances used to regulate sleep
10. Discuss the use of stimulants as a countermeasure to fatigue in the military

References

1. Smith, L., Folkard, S., Tucker, P., Macdonald, I.: Work shift duration: a review comparing eight hour and 12 hour shift systems. Occup. Environ. Med. **55**, 217–229 (1998)
2. Sack, R.L., Auckley, D., Auger, R.R., Carskadon, M.A., Wright Jr., K.P., Vitiello, M.V., Zhdanova, I.V.: Circadian rhythm sleep disorders: Part I, basic principles, shift work and jet lag disorders an American Academy of sleep medicine review. Sleep. **30**(11), 1460 (2007)
3. Brzezinski, A., Vangel, M.G., Wurtman, R.J., Norrie, G., Zhdanova, I., Ben-Shushan, A., et al.: Effects of Exogenous Melatonin on sleep: a meta-analysis. Sleep Med. Rev. **9**, 41–50 (2005)
4. Van Dongen, H., Maislin, G., Mullington, J.M., Dinges, D.F.: The cumulative cost of additional wakefulness: dose-response effects on neurobehavioral functions and sleep physiology from chronic sleep restriction and total sleep deprivation. Sleep. **26**(2), 117–126 (2003)

2

5. Waterhouse, J., Reilly, T., Atkinson, G., Edwards, B.: Jet lag: trends and coping strategies. Lancet. **369**(9567), 1117–1129 (2007). PMID 17398311. Retrieved 1 Aug 2015). https://doi.org/10.1016/S0140-6736(07)60529-7

6. Purnell, M.T., Feyer, A.-M., Herbison, G.P.: The impact of a nap performance and alertness of 12-h shift workers. J. Sleep Res. **11**(3), 219–227 (2002)

7. Caldwell, J.A., Allis, M.M., Caldwell, J.L., Paul, M.A., Miller, J.C., Neri, D.F.: Aerospace medical association aerospace fatigue countermeasures subcommittee of the human factors committee. Fatigue countermeasures in aviation. Aviat. Space Environ. Med. **80**, 29–59 (2009)

8. Taibi, D.M., Landis, L.C., Petry, H., Vitiello, M.V.: A systematic review of valerian as a sleep aid: safe but not effective. Sleep Med. Rev. **11**, 209–230 (2007)

9. Signal, L.T., Mulrine, H.M., van den Berg, M.J., Smith, A.A.T., Gander, P.H., Serfontein, W.: Mitigating and monitoring flight crew fatigue on westward ultra-long-range flight. Aviat. Space Environ. Med. **85**, 1199–1208 (2014)

10. Hursh, S.R., Raslear, T.G., Kaye, S.A., Fanzone Jr., J.F.: Validation and Calibration of a Fatigue Assessment Tool for Railroad Work Schedules, Summary Report. Department of Transportation, Washington, DC (2006). DOT/FRA/ORD-06/21, October 31, 2006

11. Brown, F.C., Buboltz, W.C., Soper, B.: Relationship of sleep hygiene awareness, sleep hygiene practices and sleep quality in university students. Behav. Med. **28**, 33–38 (2002)

12. Roach, G., Fletcher, A., Dawson, D.: A model to predict work-related fatigue based on hours of work. Aviat. Space Environ. Med. **75**(3, Section II), 61–69 (2004)

Suggested Reading by Topic

General Reference Material

Eastman, C.I., Gazda, C.J., Burgess, H.J., Crowley, S.J., Fogg, L.F.: Advancing circadian rhythms before eastward flight: a strategy to prevent or reduce jet lag. Sleep. **28**(1), 33–44 (2005)

Rajaratnam, S.M.W., Arendt, J.: Health in a 24-h society. Lancet. **358**, 999–1005 (2001)

Common Sleep Disorders

www.clevelandclinic.org/health/healthinfo/docs/3300/3373.asp?index=11429

Dinges, D.: An overview of sleepiness and accidents. J. Sleep Res. **4**(Suppl 2), 4–14 (1995)

Lamond, N., Dawson, D.: Quantifying the performance impairment associated with fatigue. J. Sleep Res. **8**, 255–262 (1999)

Leger, D.: The cost of sleep-related accidents: a report for the national commission on sleep disorders research. Sleep. **17**(1), 84–93 (1994)

Consequences of Fatigue

Blagrove, M., Alexander, C., Horne, J.A.: The effects of chronic sleep reduction on the performance of cognitive tasks sensitive to sleep deprivation. Appl. Cogn. Psychol. **9**, 21–40 (1995)

Harrison, Y., Horne, J.A.: The impact of sleep deprivation on decision making: a review. J. Exp. Psychol. **6**(3), 236–249 (2000)

Sleep Hygiene

Brown, F.C., Buboltz, W.C., Soper, B.: Relationship of sleep hygiene awareness, sleep hygiene practices and sleep quality in university students. Behav. Med. **28**, 33–38 (2002)

Purnell, M.T., Feyer, A.-M., Herbison, G.P.: The impact of a nap performance and alertness of 12-h shift workers. J. Sleep Res. **11**(3), 219–227 (2002)

Smith, L., Folkard, S., Tucker, P., Macdonald, I.: Work shift duration: a review comparing eight hour and 12 hour shift systems. Occup. Environ. Med. **55**, 217–229 (1998)

Waterhouse, J., Reilly, T., Atkinson, G., Edwards, B.: Jet lag: trends and coping strategies. Lancet. **369**(9567), 1117–1129 (2007)

General Articles Published by Aviation Agencies
UK CAA

Aircrew Fatigue: A Review of Research Undertaken on Behalf of the UK Civil Aviation Authority

EASA Flight Time Limitations (FTL) – Q&A, Aug 2015

FAA

Advisory Circular 120–100: Basics of Aviation Fatigue, June 2010

Advisory Circular 117–3: Fitness for Duty, Oct 2012

Advisory Circular 120–103A: Fatigue Risk Management Systems for Aviation Safety, May 2013

Other

Coping with long range flying. Recommendations for crew rest and alertness. Airbus, Cabon, P., et al., Nov 1995

IATA Fatigue Risk Management Guide for Airline Operators, 2nd ed., 2015

Web References

https://www.faa.gov/pilots/safety/pilotsafetybrochures/media/Fatigue_Aviation.pdf

Health and Fitness

© Springer Nature Switzerland AG 2020
E. Seedhouse et al., *Human Factors in Air Transport*,
https://doi.org/10.1007/978-3-030-13848-6_3

Learning Objectives

After completing this chapter, you should be able to

- Describe some of the ways a pilot might be incapacitated
- List some of the occupational hazards of flying
- Explain why sitting for long periods of time increases the risk of deep vein thrombosis
- List some of the benefits of exercise
- Explain how exercise can improve health and reduce occupational hazards
- List the key elements of an exercise program
- Describe some of the risks to the cardiovascular system caused by inactivity
- Explain how certain dietary practices can improve health
- List some of the psychological risks to flying
- List the elements of the IMSAFE checklist

3.1 Incapacitation Scenario

» Any condition which affects the health of a crewmember during the performance of duties which renders him or her incapable of performing the assigned duties.

  - FAA definition of incapacitation

Imagine the following scenario. You are in the right seat of a trans-Atlantic flight from Orlando to London Gatwick. A few minutes before rollback, the captain mentions he's been feeling a little queasy the past few days but feels he is fit to fly. The flight proceeds smoothly all the way to entering British airspace. Gatwick clears you through 10,000 feet and the captain asks you to make the usual requests that the cabin be prepared for landing. You glance down at the flight management system and notice you are passing the final fix as ATC instructs you to turn to a heading of 120 degrees. This instruction is not acknowledged by the captain, who appears distracted. You remind him of the ATC instruction and he corrects the turn to 160 degrees. You challenge the captain, reminding him that the ATC instruction was to turn to 120 degrees, but the captain seems unresponsive. Then he starts to shake, his body goes limp and his right leg locks and pushes the rudder, an action that causes the autopilot to disconnect. He's still semi-conscious but clearly discombobulated, evidenced by the fact that his next action is to crank on the speed!

You take control of the plane, call one of the flight attendants and ask her to get the captain out of his seat so he can be attended to. But the now-unconscious captain is a burly 250 pounds and the flight attendant can't move him, so she requests medical assistance on board. Fortunately, there are more than thirty cardiovascular surgeons onboard, all heading to the Annual Scientific Meeting for the International Society for Minimally Invasive Cardiothoracic Surgery. What are the odds? But you don't have time to ponder your good fortune as two doctors enter the cockpit and manhandle the captain to the floor. By now he is shaking violently and foaming at the mouth. The doctors start cardiopulmonary resuscitation and the captain regains consciousness. His first act is to kick the yoke, sending the aircraft into a fishtail. You ask the doctors to remove the captain from the cockpit and declare a medical emergency to ATC. A straight-in approach is granted.

Scary? Absolutely. Realistic? Ditto. Incapacitations are more common than you might think. In a six-year period in the late nineties, the FAA chalked up 39 incapacitations on board 47 aircraft. The average age was 47 with an event rate of 0.045 per 100,000 flying hours [1, 2]. The cause of all these incapacitations? Loss of consciousness, gastro-intestinal problems, neurological issues, cardiac problems. Take your pick. And the consequences? Well, if a crewmember's incapacitation results in the crew complement being reduced to below the minimum stated for that aircraft, then a PAN call must be made (some two-crew aircraft may be certified for single-pilot operations temporarily, but if an incapacitation occurs during landing when workload is increased significantly, there is little margin for error). Those are the rules. So what can be done to prevent or at least reduce the incidence of incapacitation?

3.2 Lines of Defense

Every aircraft needs maintenance, and it's no different for pilots. In fact, the rules and regulations that govern the health of pilots are just as rigorous as those that are applied to aircraft. If a pilot has a health condition, then medical certification can be delayed or denied. In some cases such a condition can cut a career short, which makes maintaining a fit and healthy lifestyle all the more important—after all, why throw away all that time and money that you spent training to become a pilot in the first place by slacking on your health and fitness?

3.3 Occupational Hazards

Pilots have stressful jobs, but it isn't just the flight planning and keeping hundreds of passengers safe that causes them stress.

3.3.1 The Dangers of Sitting

Long-term sitting can cause all sorts of problems such as back strain, disc bulge, blood pooling (◘ Fig. 3.1) herniation, clotting, abdominal distention, bloating, constipation and colon cancer. Yes, colon cancer. That is the finding of the American Cancer Society, which states quite clearly that long-term sitting contributes to colon cancer. Studies have found that men who sit for more than six hours per day had a 20% higher mortality rate than those who sat for three hours or less. More reason to stick with the regional short haul routes!

On a serious note, why does sitting down increase cancer risk? Sitting down affects your metabolism and your body's ability to assimilate glucose into the liver. The result is an elevated insulin level, which in turn accelerates *Omentum*-fat, the layer of fat more commonly referred to as "spare tire" fat. How? All that sitting down halts the activity of enzymes that have the job of breaking down lipids (i.e: fats) and for sucking up the fat out

3

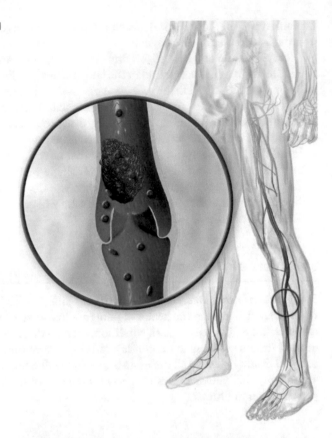

☐ **Fig. 3.1**   DVT. Credit: Medical gallery of Blausen Medical 2014

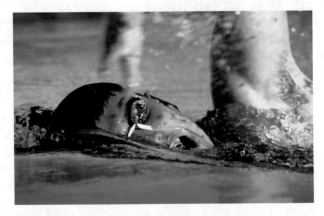

☐ **Fig. 3.2**   Swimming is a great form of exercise that can help offset all the deleterious medical effects of long-term sitting. Credit: Public domain

of our bloodstream. Sitting down for just one day in the cockpit can reduce your insulin-effectiveness by up to 40%. Multiply that by 15 workdays a month and 12 months a year and … well, you get the idea. The bottom line is that inactivity can make you insulin-resistant, and this insulin-resistance may ultimately manifest itself as Type-2 Diabetes.

What can pilots do to offset this debilitating sequence of events? Exercise (☐ Fig. 3.2)! You've got an autopilot in the cockpit. Use it. Get up out of your seat and walk around and stretch. When pilots arrive at their destination, they can use the hotel gym or go for a run. Anything to kick-start the metabolism. Dietary modification is another trick. Pilots can stick to proteins and high-fiber carbohydrates.

3.3.2 Deep Vein Thrombosis

DVT, also known as *Economy Class Syndrome*, is a scary medical condition that can kill, pure and simple. Its development is slow and insidious, meaning it creeps up on you. If you happen to be an overweight passenger or one with poor circulation and sit for hours on end in a confined space such as an economy class seat (■ Fig. 3.3), you are at risk of DVT [3, 4]. During those long hours scrunched up, there is little opportunity to move or flex your legs, which causes blood to pool in the veins until eventually a clot (thrombi) may form. This is bad because your veins are the blood vessels that return oxygen-poor blood back to the heart and lungs. When you walk, the lower leg muscles act as a pump to facilitate blood flow, but in a seated condition, that flow is impaired. Swollen ankles, hardness around the affected area, localized pressure, redness: these are all signs that a DVT may be developing. If that clot breaks loose and is circulated to the brain or the heart, then blood flow will be blocked and the result will be a stroke or an embolism. By now we are in life-threatening territory. If recognized early enough, the offending clot can be treated with aspirin, massaging and compression socks. But if you happen to be a smoker, are over 50 years old and/or have a history of cardiovascular problems, you are at even greater risk.

What can be done to reduce the risk of DVT? Given the operational risks of a passenger developing DVT (a diversion runs into the tens of thousands of dollars), it's not surprising that the problem has been very well researched. Here is what Goldhaber and Fanikos[1] recommend for passengers traveling long distances:

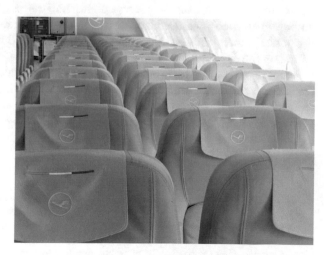

■ **Fig. 3.3** Economy class on a Lufthansa Italia Airbus A319. Credit: Felix Gottwald – ▶ www. felixgottwald.net

---

1   Adapted from Goldhaber, S.Z. & Fanikos, J. (2004). *Prevention of deep vein thrombosis and pulmonary embolism*. Journal of the American Heart Association.

3

3.3.2.1 Guidelines for Preventing DVT[2]

- Walk around the cabin every 15 to 30 minutes during flights 3 hours or longer
- Wear loose-fitting clothing, except for socks (see next item)
- Wear compression socks
- Perform simple stretching exercises while seated
- Sleep only for only 30 minutes at a time
- Limit alcohol and caffeine, since this contributes to dehydration
- Drink lots and LOTS of water
- Walk quickly through the airport during layovers
- Note: for people with cardiovascular diseases, heparin (a blood thinner) may work

3.3.2.2 Suggested Inflight Exercises to Prevent DVT[3]

- Foot lifts. Alternate keeping toes on the floor and lifting heels with keeping heels on the floor and lifting your toes
- Knee lifts. Sitting straight up, keep knees bent and lift thigh. Alternate legs
- Toe curls. Curl toes and release. Press toes down against the floor or just wiggle inside your shoes
- Ankle rotations. Lift feet off the floor and draw a circle with toes, trying to get a full range of ankle motion. Repeat in the opposite direction

3.3.3 Sinusitis

Today's airliners circulate much higher quality air than aircraft just ten years ago. For example, the Airbus only recirculates half its air, with the remainder being engine-inlet, high-pressure bleed air. To make this air as breathable as possible for the passengers, it is filtered through HEPA filters, but this process still leaves the air a little on the dry side. And when you're breathing dry air for hours on end, sinusitis can be the outcome. The problem with conditioning air, as all airliners do, is that the air has almost no humidity, which is not surprising because that air is taken from cruise altitude at around 35,000 feet, where the air tends to be cold and dry. Dry air is very tough on the mucus membrane lining the sinuses, which quickly dry out.

---

2   Adapted from: FAA Travel Brochure *Deep Vein Thrombosis and Travel*.
3   Another study published by the same journal, examined 21 years of general aviation incidents between 1983 and 2003. In this period, 37 pilots either attempted or committed suicide by aircraft. More than a dozen of the pilots had psychiatric problems.

3.3.4 **Back Pain**

Of all the myriad occupational health hazards faced by pilots, back pain (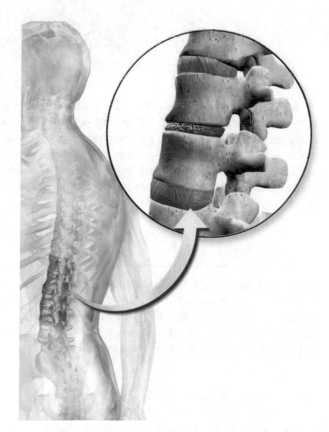 Fig. 3.4) is one of the most prevalent. A pilot doesn't have to have a back problem to have back pain—sitting in a pilot's seat for eight hours is enough to make anyone suffer back trouble [5]. The spine comprises three support curves: the cervical, thoracic and the lumbar. These curves are designed to distribute your upper-body weight and also to provide you with spinal flexibility. For most activities, the spine works well, but sitting down for extended periods results in excessive weight being supported by the lumbar area. This in turn puts a great strain on the intervertebral lumbar discs of cartilage and also the surrounding ligaments. And if you happen to have poor posture, which is difficult to avoid after sitting for six or seven plus hours, then back pain is the consequence. Repeat extended periods of sitting over several months and years and the result is chronic back pain that may ultimately manifest itself as a slipped disc, a herniated disc or perhaps nerve damage. Excruciating pain follows, and often the only solution is surgery. Twinges? Shooting pain down your legs? Bouts of tingling or numbness in your back? Chances are you have a lower back pain (LBP) condition.

Fig. 3.4 Back pain can be caused by the vertebrae compressing the intervertebral discs. Credit: Medical gallery of Blausen Medical 2014

3

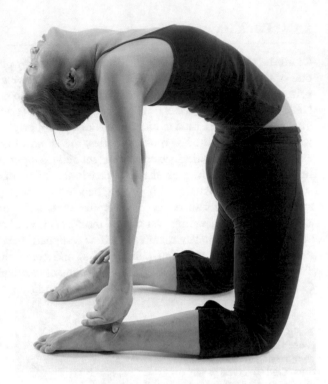

◪ **Fig. 3.5**   The *Ustrasana*, also known as the camel pose, is one of several yoga asana poses. Credit: OrenBochman

So what can pilots do to reduce the chances of experiencing back pain? They can help themselves by getting up and moving around every once in a while, they can practice yoga (◪ Fig. 3.5) at home, and they can adjust those lumbar supports found in so many airline seats nowadays—the key is to adjust the support *forward* and *up* so the inward lumbar curve is supported. By doing this, the weight of the upper body is placed on the pelvis [6]. And when pilots travel to and from their work, they should exercise effective body mechanics when lifting.

3.4   Exercise

A common theme when talking about all the health problems faced by pilots is exercise, as not only is it the perfect countermeasure to so many of today's illnesses and ailments, but it is also the foundation of a healthy life generally (Appendix III). There are literally thousands and thousands of studies that support the role of regular exercise in decreasing the risk of disease. But what constitutes exercise?

3.4.1   Exercise Workouts

Pilots are busy, so they need a workout that is short but effective, such as the 5BX. Developed by the Royal Canadian Air Force a while back, the 5BX comprises just five basic exercises, hence its name. A bestseller back in the 1960s and 1970s (it sold 23 million copies around the world), the 5BX has stood the test of time partly because it is simple and effective. The plan has six charts organized in increasing order of difficulty. Each of the charts includes the same five exercises that take 11 minutes to perform. The first four exercises include stretching, sit-ups, back extensions, and pushups, while the fifth exercise is aerobic exercise. As the person performing the routine progresses, the number and difficulty of each type of exercise increases.

3.4.2 Elements of an Exercise Program

The 5BX is one example of a short exercise routine that includes the key elements of an exercise program, which we'll discuss here.
1. Warm-up
2. Flexibility
3. Aerobic Conditioning
4. Anaerobic Conditioning
5. Cool-Down

First, the warm-up. This should be specific to the type of exercise you're planning. The warm-up, which can include light jogging, helps prime your body for the exercise routine by delivering more oxygen to the muscles. After some light jogging, it is a good idea to include some stretching to increase muscle and joint flexibility and to reduce the risk of injury while performing the actual routine. Next, the aerobic element of the workout. Aerobic exercise is any exercise—swimming, cycling, running—that forces the cardiovascular system to work and that includes the large muscle groups. The aerobic component should be followed by an anaerobic session that can target a particular muscle group or groups. This type of training in more intense and can include free weights and resistance machines. Finally, the routine should be completed by a cool-down, which comprises low-intensity exercise similar to that used for the warm-up.

3.4.3 Benefits of Exercise

There are hundreds of books that detail the benefits of exercise. What follows is a snapshot of the main points.
1. A regular exercise routine (i.e: at least three times per week for at least 20 minutes per session) helps control weight.
2. It helps manage blood sugar levels, because regular exercise helps your body utilize insulin more effectively. This can reduce the risk of type 2 diabetes.
3. Regular exercise can help smokers quit the habit by reducing withdrawal symptoms.
4. During exercise, your body releases chemicals that make you feel more relaxed, which can help a person better deal with stress.
5. Cognitive reasoning is improved by exercise, because it stimulates the body to release chemicals that help enhance learning and judgment.

3

6. Stronger bones and muscles are a direct result of a regular exercise routine. Running is especially helpful in building good bone density and strength.
7. Want to reduce the risk of certain cancers? Regular exercise is the answer. Hundreds of peer-reviewed research papers have demonstrated the protective effect exercise has in reducing the risk of colon, uterine and lung cancer.
8. Have trouble sleeping? Exercise helps you fall asleep faster and stay asleep longer.
9. Cardiovascular disease. Yes, regular exercise is a powerful risk reducer when it comes to cardiovascular disease. Exercise promotes blood flow, which in turn increases oxygen flow to all parts of the body.
10. Longer lifespan. Again, there are hundreds of peer-reviewed research papers showing that exercise can increase your chances of living longer by reducing the risk of certain cancers and heart disease.

3.5 Cardiovascular Health

One of the many reasons working as an airline pilot is such a risky occupation is because it constitutes shift work. Those who work shifts are more prone to all sorts of medical conditions, the most common being cardiovascular problems [7]. In a recent *British Medical Journal* study, it was reported that shift work increased the risk of having a heart attack by 23% and the risk of having a coronary event by 24%. Fortunately, while cardiovascular disease is common in the aviation world, having a cardiovascular problem (◘ Fig. 3.6) does not mean a pilot will be grounded, since the FAA is able to issue waivers for certain conditions (it issues about 5,000 to 6,000 Special Issuance Authorizations every year). In fact, only one tenth of a percent of all medical applications are denied outright. According to ALPA, 23% of the pilots that contact the association do so for cardiovascular conditions. The most common condition is myocardial infarction (Aside), more commonly known as a heart attack. Other common conditions include atrial fibrillation, hypertension, valvular disease and arrhythmias.

◘ **Fig. 3.6** Illustration depicting atherosclerosis in a coronary artery. Credit: Medical gallery of Blausen Medical 2014

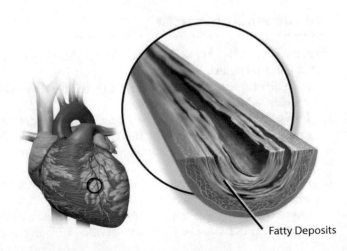

Fatty Deposits

A Heart Attack

What happens to a pilot who suffers a heart attack? First and foremost, this will mean a trip to the emergency room. A cardiologist will be called and the pilot—let's call him Bob—will be rushed to the cardiac catheterization laboratory ("cath lab" for short) for an angiogram. The angiogram will determine if Bob's coronary artery is blocked. If it is, Bob may undergo a procedure in the cath lab performed by a cardiologist. Most likely, this procedure will be a percutaneous transluminal coronary angioplasty (PTCA), which involves inflating a balloon inside the coronary artery to squash the cholesterol plaque off the artery and allow blood to flow again. If the condition is worse, Bob might have to undergo coronary artery bypass grafting. In either case, Bob's chances of continuing as a pilot are not good, because myocardial infarction and coronary artery disease are two disqualifying conditions in the eyes of the FAA. Having said that, Bob has a chance by applying for a waiver via the special issuance process (14 CFR 67.401).

How does the FAA treat these disorders? For heart rhythm disorders it can issue certificates depending on the nature of the underlying disease. For example, heart murmurs are evaluated on a 1 to 6 scale. On the low end of the scale, a medical clearance is likely, but at the high end of the scale, a medical investigation must be performed, which may include a monitoring period. For other conditions such as atrial fibrillation, pilots must be tested and treated, but for conditions such as left bundle branch block (a heart signal abnormality), frequent evaluation will most likely be necessary. At the riskier end of the scale of cardiovascular problems are conditions such as sudden cardiac arrest, a stroke with associated neurocognitive impairment, and having an implantable cardiac defibrillator fitted; each of these is cause for denial of a medical certificate.

3.6 Diet

Pilots are meticulous when it comes to the airworthiness of their aircraft, but do they exercise and apply the same care when it comes to looking after their health and their diet (◘ Fig. 3.7) in particular? Next time you are waiting at a gate, take a look at the aircrew and pay particular attention to their waistlines. Then revisit that question. While the majority of pilots eat healthy, there are some who would do well to improve their eating habits. But what is the best way for pilots to eat?

Scientists at the University of North Dakota reckon they have the answer. In a 2009 study, Dr. Glenda and Dr. Paul Lindseth performed a study of pilots regarding how particular diets affected flight performance. The participants in the study were randomly assigned to one of three diets, one being high in fat, a second high in carbohydrate, and the third high in protein. After some time on their assigned diet, the participants' flight performance was assessed in a full-motion simulator. In addition to being evaluated in the simulator, the participants were required to perform various cognitive function tests. The news was not so good for high-protein aficionados. The participants who followed the high-fat and high-carbohydrate diets performed significantly better than those who followed the high protein diet. Worse for the high-protein group was that these participants reported higher than normal anxiety levels and sleepless-

3

Fig. 3.7 A selection of plant-sourced food consumed by humans. Credit: Agricultural Research Service, the research agency of the United States Department of Agriculture/ID K11083–1

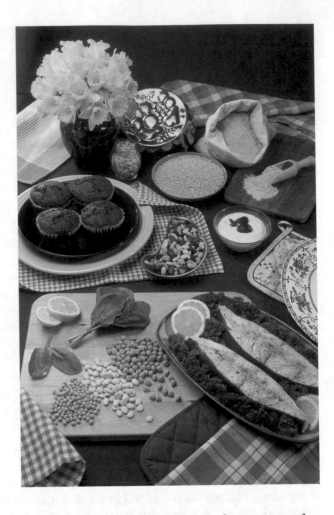

ness. The pattern of performance was similar when the participants' cognitive performance tests were evaluated. Response times (assessed by applying the Sternberg Test of Mental Agility) for the high-fat dieters were significantly faster than those on the high-protein diet.

» These study results contribute significantly to our understanding of the effects diet can have on cognition and performance. With additional research, these findings may help decrease the number of aviation accidents due to pilot error.

  - Dr. Glenda Lindseth

So diet affects cognitive function and flight performance, but what about the practical applications of the UND study for pilots? Pilots should reduce their intake of processed foods and sugars and also ensure their carbohydrate and fat intake is greater than their protein intake. For those who take a deeper interest in their diet and performance, it is helpful to understand the effect of certain nutrients such as the essential amino acids. A lack of any one of these can affect cognitive and overall performance (Aside).

Chemicals that affect sleep and wakefulness

Tyrosine is a non-essential amino acid that helps increase alertness, while tryptophan is an essential amino acid that does the opposite. Serotonin on the other hand is derived from tryptophan, but its effect is to promote a feeling of wellbeing. Then there is dopamine, which has all sorts of functions related to mood, sleep and learning. This sort of information is useful for a pilot traveling across time zones. At the beginning of the day, it obviously makes sense to eat foods that will increase tyrosine (proteins and minimal carbohydrates) levels, while at the end of the day it makes sense to eat foods that will boost tryptophan (protein, carbohydrates) levels and promote sleep.

3.7 Mental Health

In a study published in the *Journal of Environmental Health*, 13% of airline pilots met the criteria for clinical depression. Think about that next time you're taxiing for takeoff! In that same study it was reported that 4% of airline pilots admitted to having suicidal thoughts within two weeks of taking the survey [8]. Did the Journal of Environmental Health get their metrics correct? The study—to which 1,500 pilots responded—used a depression questionnaire known as PHQ-9, and the statistics were no different than those found in the general population. But because these are pilots we are talking about, the media jumped all over it. And the media did what it does best: they took scientific results, dumbed them down, distorted them, embellished them and then sensationalized the story in their unique sound-bite style. People lapped it up, and why not? After all, the story of the Germanwings pilot's suicide crash (Aside) was still fresh in many people's minds.

The case of Andreas Lubitz: Germanwings Flight 9525

On March 24, 2015, Germanwings Flight 9525 departed Barcelona en-route to Düsseldorf. The aircraft, an Airbus A320-211, was 100 km northwest of Nice when it crashed into a mountainside (◘ Fig. 3.8). All 144 passengers and six crew were killed. The copilot, Andreas Lubitz, had been declared unfit for work by a doctor who had treated Lubitz for suicidal tendencies. Lubitz disregarded the doctor's recommendation and reported for work. After the aircraft reached cruise altitude, the captain left the cockpit. Lubitz then locked the cockpit door and plunged the aircraft into a controlled descent while alarmed passengers looked on in horror. Attempts by French air traffic to contact Germanwings Flight 9525 were unsuccessful, so a French (military) Mirage jet was deployed to intercept the errant Airbus, but it was too late.

The investigation into the incident revealed Lubitz had been taking prescription drugs. Searches on the copilot's computer indicated Lubitz had searched for "ways to commit suicide" and "cockpit doors and their security provisions". The prosecutor in the case reported that doctors had informed Lubitz that he should not have been flying, but due to German secrecy regulations, this medical information could not be provided to Germanwings. In response to the tragedy, some aviation authorities implemented new regulations that required two crewmembers in the cockpit at all times, a regulation that had been in place for years in the United States. There was also a call to improve support in the psychological testing and monitoring of pilots.

3

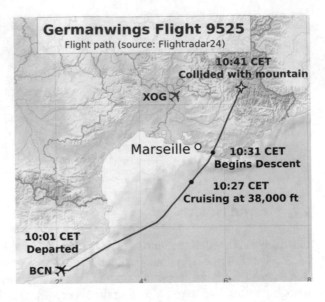

》 I really wish that we had some kind of deeper thinking about this issue, because it's one of the most difficult in aviation medicine.

- Alpo Vuorio, MD, PhD, aviation specialist in occupational medicine at the Mehiläinen Airport Health Centre, Finland

Sadly, Andreas Lubitz was not the first pilot to commit suicide by aircraft. In a study published in the *Journal of Aviation, Space and Environmental Medicine* in 2014, scientists examined 20 years of flight data between 1993 and 2012 and found that 24 of 7,244 aircraft crashes were thought to have been caused by pilots deliberately crashing the aircraft [1]. That figure represents less than one percent of the total, but it is still cause for concern. The Germanwings incident was first and foremost the result of the failure of the system—a system that requires little or no psychological screening for those charged with $250 million aircraft and the lives of hundreds of passengers. In the United States, pilots must undergo medical evaluations once or twice a year depending on their age. The medical certificate that is issued by an FAA-certified doctor reflects the physical health of the pilot, but it does not reflect a psychological evaluation. Unlike some professions such as astronauts, pilots are more or less immune from having to be subjected to rigorous psychological testing, which, given the responsibility pilots have, is concerning. While the FAA allows pilots to take certain antidepressants, this is a flimsy safeguard. Obviously it is impossible to bulletproof any profession against every human weakness, but extensive psychological testing combined with a yearly psychiatric evaluation would seem to be a good start.

》 Pilots aren't going to tell you anything, any more than a medical doctor would about their mental health. The problem is there is no incentive to report mental health issues. They know that if they self report, the way the system is designed, it will be a black mark.

- Scott Shappell, professor, Human Factors Department, Embry-Riddle Aeronautics University

Scott is right. Pilots are unlikely to report mental health problems, because they know that if they do they will be taken out of the sky [9]. And the medical doctors who sign the medical certification every year are not always qualified to detect all mental health problems. This is a problem. According to Dr. William Sledge, a physician who has assessed pilots for the FAA, about one third of the group he evaluated reported mental health problems such as anxiety. Compounding the problem was the fact that only half of Dr. Sledge's group reported their problems (the remaining pilots were referred after superiors intervened).

>> Pilots must disclose all existing physical and psychological conditions and medications or face significant fines of up to $250,000 if they are found to have falsified information.

- FAA statement on pilot's mental health

Does extra screening and/or mental health screening actually work? In 1995 the US Air Force implemented required suicide prevention and awareness training, a program that included screening for mental health issues. The result? The USAF suicide rate fell from 16 suicides per 100,000 members to 9.

On March 27, 2012, JetBlue Flight 191 captain Clayton Osborn snapped. This was a problem because at the time of his meltdown, the Airbus A-320 was flying from New York to Las Vegas. Osborn began what some passengers described as a panic attack, shouting al Qaeda threats and using the words "bomb", "Iran" and "Iraq". Eventually, he was subdued by passengers and the co-pilot took over.

>> What I actually witnessed was a radical pilot trying to break into the cockpit. I think that the copilot changed the codes for him to get back in. The pilot started banging on the door to let him in. "Why did you change the code? We got to drop this plane to 7,000 feet". It appeared that's what he wanted to do—open up the side door. He wanted to open up that side door.

- David Gonzalez, explaining to Fox News how he subdued JetBlue pilot Clayton Osborn

3.7.1 Assessing Mental Health

Under FAA regulations, pilots must undergo a medical exam every six or 12 months depending on age. This exam must be conducted by an Aviation Medical Examiner (AME). The FAA medical form includes questions on mental health, and if pilots do not disclose this information they face fines. While certain conditions such as bipolar disorder or psychosis will disqualify a pilot from FAA medical certification, other conditions can be treated. Many airlines have implemented reporting and monitoring programs to help pilots report any mental health condition.

3.8 The IMSAFE Checklist

How do airlines assess whether a pilot is healthy enough to fly? In short, they can't. There is no black and white measure of how stressed a pilot is, and there are no formal regulations in place that state how much each pilot should exercise and what

3

types of foods they should eat. But there are plenty of checklists in the aviation world: climb checklists, emergency checklists, takeoff checklists, startup checklists. The list of checklists goes on and on. So it isn't surprising that there is a checklist for determining fitness to fly. The FAA calls it the I M S A F E checklist (Appendix IV) and here it is:

- **I – Illness**: Every pilot should ask if they are healthy, and if not, if flying anyway will put lives at risk. For example, if a pilot has a cold, then the change in cabin pressure may cause problems during descent or ascent.
- **M – Medication**: Some medications can be used by pilots, and some can't. It's up to the pilot to check if the medication they are using is on the prohibited list.
- **S – Stress**: This is a difficult one because a pilot can feel fine, but if they have been under a lot of stress then performance can be affected.
- **A – Alcohol**: This is a "No-No". Alcohol reduces reaction time, impairs judgment and affects vision. That's why the FAA has a rule stating that a pilot cannot fly within eight hours of drinking alcohol or with a blood content that exceeds 0.04%.
- **F – Fatigue**: Another difficult one. What is a metric for fatigue? How can it be measured? A combination of resting heart rate, blood pressure and quality of sleep is a start, but the FAA has not implemented a fatigue metric. So it's up to the pilots to judge for themselves if they are too fatigued to fly.
- **E – Emotion**: Depressed? Anxious? Emotionally stable? If a pilot answers "no" to all three questions, then perhaps they should reconsider flying.

3.9 **Summary**

Human physiology is an increasingly significant topic in the aviation safety arena due to the aging population and the trend of longer and longer flights. Furthermore, the hazards of cardiovascular disease may be compounded by these two factors, with the result that DVT is now a serious issue facing airlines. Another worrying trend is the psychological state of pilots and the fact that there is no assessment of this in the selection procedure. Since the Andreas Lubitz incident, there have been several other "suicide by aircraft" incidents, which has prompted an increased human factors emphasis on this aspect of mental illness.

Key Terms
AME - Aviation Medical Examiner

DVT - Deep Vein Thrombosis

IMSAFE - Illness, Medication, Stress, Alcohol, Fatigue, Eating

PTLA - Percutaneous Transluminal Coronary Angioplasty

Review Questions
1. Explain what is meant by DVT
2. List 5 key elements of an exercise program
3. What is a Special Issuance Authorization, and under what circumstances might one be applied?
4. List 3 hazards of sitting for long periods
5. What are tyrosine and tryptophan?
6. Explain how the risk of DVT might be reduced
7. List 5 benefits of a regular exercise program
8. What is the IMSAFE checklist?
9. How do fat, protein and carbohydrate affect reaction times in pilots?
10. Who was Andreas Lubitz?

References

1. Feijó, D., Luiz, R.R., Camara, V.M.: Common mental disorders among civil aviation pilots. Aviat. Space Environ. Med. **83**(5), 509–513 (2012)
2. Cooper, C., Sloan, S.: Occupational and psychological stress among commercial airline pilots. J. Occup. Med. **27**, 570–576 (1985)
3. Bagshaw, M.: Traveler's thrombosis: a review of deep vein thrombosis associated with travel. The Air Transport Medicine Committee of the Aerospace Medical Association. Aviat. Space Environ. Med. **72**, 848–851 (2001)
4. Cruikshank, J.M., Gorlin, R., Janett, B.: Air travel and thrombotic episode: the economy class syndrome. Lancet. **II**, 497–498 (1988)
5. Froom, P., Barzilay, S., Caine, Y., Margaliot, S., Forecast, D.: Low back pain in pilots. Aviat. Space Environ. Med. **57**(7), 694–695 (1986)
6. Landau, D.A., Chapnick, L., Yoffe, N., Azaria, B., Goldstein, L., Atar, E.: Cervical and lumbar MRI findings in aviators as a function of aircraft type. Aviat. Space Environ. Med. **77**(11), 1158–1161 (2006)
7. Ryan, T.J., et al.: Patients with acute myocardial infarction. A report of the American College of Cardiology/American Heart Association Task Force on Practice Guidelines. Circulation. **100**, 1016–1030 (1999)
8. Sanne, B., Mykletun, A., Dahl, A.A., Moen, B.E., Tell, G.S.: Occupational differences in levels of anxiety and depression: the Hordaland health study. J. Occup. Environ. Med. **45**(6), 628–638 (2003)
9. Koonce, J.M.: A brief history of aviation psychology. Hum. Factors. **26**(5), 499–508 (1984)

Suggested Reading

https://www.faa.gov/pilots/safety/pilotsafetybrochures/media/MedCertforWeb.pdf
https://www.leftseat.com/special_issuance.htm

Vision

© Springer Nature Switzerland AG 2020
E. Seedhouse et al., *Human Factors in Air Transport*,
https://doi.org/10.1007/978-3-030-13848-6_4

Learning Objectives
After completing this chapter, you should be able to
- Describe the basic anatomy of the eye
- Explain the impact that night has on a pilot's vision
- Distinguish between photopic and scotopic vision
- Explain what is meant by visual acuity and what is meant by 20/20 vision
- Explain what is meant by depth perception
- Discuss the limitations of someone with myopia, hyperopia and presbyopia
- Describe the primary somatogyral illusions
- Distinguish between the primary runway illusions
- Describe some of the vision issues that may be encountered in later life, with specific reference to cataracts
- Explain how aviation illusions can be prevented

4.1 Introduction

Flying is especially demanding on vision, for the simple reason that humans are not physiologically designed to operate at high speeds in three-dimensional space. It is because of the limitations of human vision that pilots are susceptible to illusions and have problems flying at night.

4.2 Eye Physiology

Most pilots have a basic knowledge of the optical characteristics of the eye, since before they start flying they need to know what their uncorrected vision is and if they have any general visual problems. But vision is much, much more than whether a pilot is far-sighted or nearsighted. The process of *seeing* comprises a spectrum of events that starts with the transmission of light energy from the cornea and ends with the processing of that information in the brain.

4.2.1 Anatomy of the Eye

The basic anatomy of the eye is depicted in ◻ Fig. 4.1. Light enters the eye through the cornea and passes through the pupil. The amount of light entering can be controlled by either dilating or constricting the pupil, a function that is taken care of by the iris (the colored part of the eye). The pupil functions in a very similar way to the diaphragm of a camera because it controls the amount of light entering the eye. Once light has passed through the pupil it must be focused, and this is where the lens comes into play. The lens focuses light onto the surface of the retina, which is the eyeball's inner layer. Lined with photosensitive cells called rods and cones, it is the retina that actually records the image. The region of sharpest vision—the macula—is located in the center of the retina, where

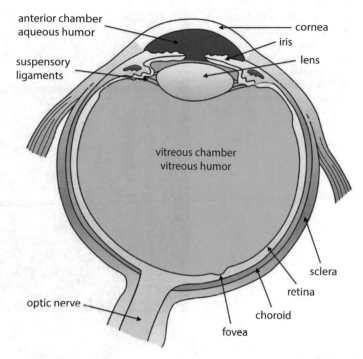

Fig. 4.1 The structures of the eye labelled. Credit: Holly Fischer (► http://open.umich.edu/education/med/resources/second-look-series/materials)

the concentration of cones is at its highest. In fact, at the very center of the macula, a depression called the fovea contains only cones. In addition to being used for high-intensity day vision, the cones help us with central vision to determine detail and color and identify distant objects.

4.2.2 Rod, Cones and Blind Spots

The rods on the other hand are located mainly around the retina (**Fig. 4.2**). The rods are used in low light conditions and with night vision and to help us with peripheral vision and detection of position references that may be fixed or moving. The rods operate in shades of gray and are not used to determine detail or perceive color. Another important feature of the retina is located at the back of the eye at the junction of the optic nerve and the optic disc. This area is devoid of rods and cones, therefore the eye is blind in this spot. This isn't normally a problem because the eyes compensate thanks to our binocular vision, but if our field of vision (FoV) is obstructed by an object such as oncoming aircraft, that object could fall in the blind spot and go undetected. Another blind spot is the Night Blind Spot, which appears in low light conditions as a result of there being no rods in the fovea. Just 5 to 10 degrees wide in the center of your FoV, this particular blind spot may appear as a result of viewing an object directly at night—the object in this case would go undetected.

4

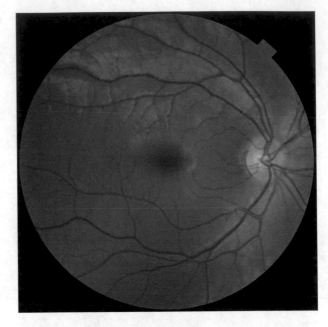

■ **Fig. 4.2** Fundus photograph showing the blood vessels in a normal human retina. Veins are darker and slightly wider than corresponding arteries. The optic disc is at right, and the macula lutea is near the center. Credit: Medical gallery of Mikael Häggström 2014

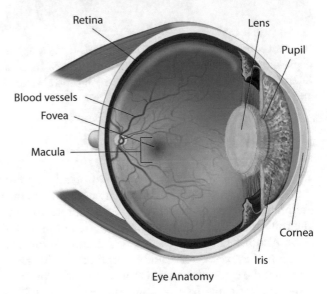

■ **Fig. 4.3** Illustration showing main structures of the eye including the fovea. Credit: Medical gallery of Blausen Medical 2014

4.2.3   The Fovea

This feature (■ Fig. 4.3), which sits in the center of the macula, contains a high concentration of cones but no rods. It is this area where our vision is at its sharpest. But it is a very narrow part of our vision. To put foveal vision in perspective, consider that the FoV of each eye is 135° vertically and 160° horizontally. Foveal FoV represents just 1°. That's small. Really small. How small is 1°? Take out a quarter and tape it to a window. Now step back 4.5 feet and close one eye. The area of your FoV covered by the quarter is a 1° field—in other words, similar to your foveal vision. But why is this important to pilots? Well, because the amount of detail a pilot can see outside of that foveal FoV is actually quite small. Outside of a 10° cone that is concentric to the foveal 1° cone, a pilot can see one tenth of what he or she sees within the foveal FoV. So, if a pilot is able to see an oncoming aircraft at 5,000 feet away using foveal FoV, that same aircraft wouldn't be detected using peripheral vision until it was just 500 feet away! This is the reason that flight instructors badger their students to keep scanning.

4.3 Vision Modes

Thanks to us having such a versatile vision system, we can operate very well across a range of luminance levels; it's just a case of utilizing the right equipment for the job. Let's begin with daytime vision.

4.3.1 Photopic Vision

During the day we rely on central vision, which is enabled by the foveal cones. These allow us to perceive and interpret sharp images and colors.

4.3.2 Mesopic Vision

When light levels fall, as they do during dusk and dawn, we humans switch to *mesopic* vision, which is enabled thanks to the use of central vision and the peripheral rods.

4.3.3 Night Vision

Night vision, which is also known as *scotopic vision*, can only be used once dark adaptation has taken place. This process is dependent on the rods and the cones, both of which contain photopigments that are key to the process by which eyes increase their sensitivity to darkness. On exposure to low levels of illumination, the photopigments regenerate until retinal sensitivity reaches its maximum level. For the rods, 20 to 30 minutes is required for this process to be complete, whereas the cones reach maximum sensitivity after only five or six minutes. The problem is that if, after having adapted to the dark, the eyes are exposed to bright light of sufficient duration (more than one second), retinal sensitivity is impaired and the process has to start all over again. In the world of aviation, dark adaptation is critical for night operations, which is why red light is used to illuminate the cockpit. Why red? Red light has a wavelength less than 650 nanometers, and the rods are not sensitive to light greater than this wavelength. The problem with red lighting is that it creates near-vision problems, which is why low level white lighting is more commonly used.

4.3.4 Accommodation Time

This is simply the time it takes for your eye to adjust the focal length to the distance of an object you are looking at. This time is important in flying because large accommodations are required between those objects you see outside the cockpit and the instruments inside the cockpit. For example, the time it takes from scanning for objects outside to checking a reading on an instrument panel is about 2.4 seconds. For an average airliner at cruise speed, you would travel about one third of a mile in that time. Accommodation time increases as you get older and is also affected by light intensity.

4.3.5 Visual Acuity

Visual acuity is a measure of your vision system's capacity for spatial resolving. In other words, it is your ability to distinguish between small objects at distance and also to distinguish contrasts. The degree to which you can spatially resolve is determined by factors such as refractive errors, aberrations, illumination and contrast. Another factor is the relative motion between the object you are trying to fixate on and you. This factor is determined by *ocular pursuit*, which is capable of maintaining a steady fixation on an object at an angular velocity below 30° per second.

4.3.6 Depth Perception

This feature of your vision is determined by your brain's ability to judge the relative distance of objects and the spatial relationship of objects at distance. To do this, your brain relies on two binocular cues known as *vergence* (convergence) and *stereopsis*.

— **Vergence** is basically the degree with which your eyes have to rotate to place the images of the objects you want to observe on the foveas. The degree of convergence depends on the distance to the object being observed: the closer the object is to you, the greater the degree of convergence.

— **Stereopsis** on the other hand is a function of the separation between your eyes, which happens to be about 6 cm. This interpupillary separation—a feature known as *retinal disparity*—results in each eye viewing an object slightly differently. So, if you are viewing two objects at different distances, each of those objects will be viewed at a different binocular angle. The way the brain processes the information and combines the views of two or more objects is the process of stereopsis.

These characteristics of depth perception become important during approach and landing, because the most important cues (runway size for example) for spatial orientation during this phase happen to be some distance away. This affects depth perception because of the way the eyes work during stereopsis.

4.4 Factors Affecting Vision

As versatile and capable as our vision system is, there are a number of ways it can be affected (◘ Fig. 4.4): ambient illumination, atmospheric clarity, smoke, fog, dust in the air... the list goes on and on. Generally, the bigger the object, the better the illumination, the better the contrast and the longer viewing time, the better the visibility. But at night the identification of objects is degraded substantially, simply because our vision system doesn't work as well as it does during the day.

Even during the day there are factors that can conspire to make life difficult for pilots. Surface references or the horizon can be obscured by smog, haze, fog or a combination of these factors. Equally, excessive ambient illumination can be a headache for a pilot. Lack of features can also strain your eyes, as can glare caused by clouds, snow or water. Flying over terrain that causes glare can result in squinting and even temporary blindness. Then there are the effects of self-imposed stresses such as alcohol, smoking, hypoglycemia and sleep deprivation, all of which can seriously degrade vision. Smokers for example, are more susceptible to hypoxia than non-smokers. In addition to smoking, the self-imposed stresses of self-medication, alcohol consumption, hypoglycemia, sleep deprivation and excessive fatigue can all conspire to seriously impair vision. Then there are problems such as windscreen haze, scratched windshields, inadequate cockpit environmental controls, improper cockpit illumination, sustained visual workload, altitude and color vision [1–3]. We'll take a closer look at the latter two here.

4.4.1 Altitude

One of the first senses to be affected by lack of oxygen is our vision. Color vision begins to deteriorate between 1,500 to 3,300 meters, and night vision may be impaired at altitudes as low as 1,500 m. Higher than 5,000 m and visual effects become very pronounced since accommodation and convergence are affected, with the result that pilots may experience double vision.

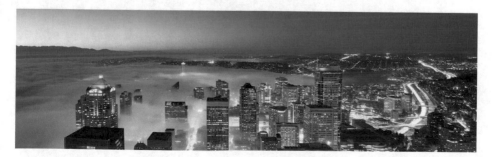

◘ Fig. 4.4 Fog rolls into Seattle from the sea. Credit: Patrick Rodriguez

4.4.2 **Color Vision**

About 8% of males and half a percent of females have color perception problems [3]. The medical standards in FAR Part 67 state applicants for all classes of aviation medical certification shall have "the ability to perceive those colors necessary for the safe performance of airman duties".

Determining whether an applicant meets this requirement is usually achieved using the pseudoisochromatic color plate test (◘ Fig. 4.5). If you fail the test, you can still fly, but there are limits—one of which is no night flying, which means you won't be able to get a job with the airlines. Okay, that's not quite true. If you're not happy being limited to flying during the day, you can request an alternative color plate test such as the Dvorine second edition 15-plate test. If you pass one of these alternative color tests, the FAA will consider your vision as meeting the standards set in FAR Part 67. For Class I medicals, you will also need to pass an operational color vision test (OCVT) and a color vision medical test, which is a flight test.

4.4.2.1 **Tallahassee B727 Accident: Copilot Color Vision Deficiency**

Aircraft accidents in which color perception defects have been cited as a contributing factor are rare but have occurred. One example is the crash of FedEx flight 1478 (a Boeing 727) in Tallahassee in 2002 during a night visual approach. In this case, the first officer's color deficiency interfered with his ability to discern the red and white lights of the PAPI.

The crew of FedEx Flight 1478 survived and gave evidence to the NTSB. The copilot who was flying the aircraft had a color vision defect. The Captain and the Second Officer had normal color vision. None of the crew noticed the danger of crashing short of the

◘ **Fig. 4.5**   Ishihara Plate No. 1 (12). Credit: Nicoguaro

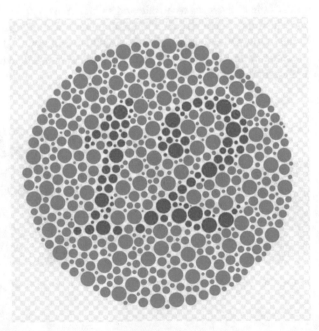

runway, although this should have been apparent to them from the PAPI lights. Although fatigue was deemed to have been a significant factor in regards to the performance of the Captain and the First Officer, the NTSB's report indicated that the major cause of the crash was the copilot's defective vision. The NTSB, which recommended to the FAA that stricter color vision screening be implemented for aircrew, made no mention of the design features of the PAPI system. This is of interest because the aircrew that had no color vision defect failed to process the information presented to them by the PAPI system. The cause of the Flight 1478 accident was foreshadowed all the way back in 1981 in a paper (*Hazards of Color Coding in Visual Approach Slope Indicators*) by Clark and Gordon. Published by the Department of Defense Aeronautical Research Laboratories, the paper concluded:

» Color coding as a primary cue is almost universally condemned in the ergonomics literature and an examination in this report of the numerous factors which act to degrade the reliability of color-coded primary signals from VASI's supports the view that <u>neither Red-White VASIS nor PAPI should be used in air transport operations</u>. Apart from reasonably common circumstances which render color-coded signals from these aids as unreliable, e.g. atmospheric conditions and windshield and projection optics scattering, there is a strong prima facie case that the signals, through combinations of physical and physiological circumstances which are not rare, <u>can become sufficiently misleading as to be hazardous</u>.

Despite the warning flags, Australia was forced by the ICAO to adopt PAPI instead of significantly safer T-VASIS system, which used shape coding as primary slope guidance. PAPI was cheaper, and in this case cost considerations won out over safety.

Studies of color perception in the aviation environment have so far been limited. Further research in this area is required to determine precisely the importance of color perception and what defects can be allowed without affecting safety.

4.5 Aviation Illusions

» Saddam had exploded the oil rigs to fill the air with oil. I couldn't see the Cobra in front of me or the stars or the moon. It was just black.

- Major Paul "Goose" Gosden, US Marine Corps, describing flying through an oil cloud as night during the second Gulf War

Military pilots spend an extraordinary amount of time training to fly at night. But flying through an oil cloud at night adds another level of complexity to what is already a demanding task. Not convinced? OK. Do you have an XBox? Great. Now load the helicopter combat game *Apache*, fly over enemy territory—at night, remember—and then turn off the television but *not* the XBox and try to land blind. Not so easy is it? That's because you're experiencing *spatial disorientation*, which is exactly what Gosden was going through. Spatial disorientation (◘ Fig. 4.6) [4, 5] is a broad term that includes all sorts of illusions, and the one that Gosden was experiencing was *the leans*. We'll return to this type of illusion in a moment, but first a reminder of how pilots fly.

4

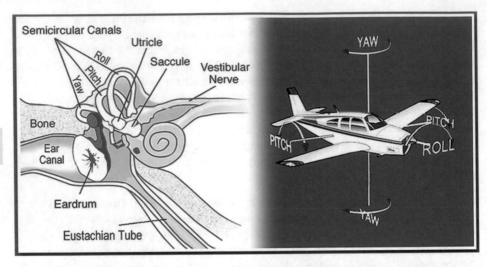

Fig. 4.6 The inner ear with semicircular canals shown, likening them to the roll, pitch and yaw axis of an aircraft. Credit: ▶ http://www.cami.jccbi.gov/aam-400/phys_intro.htm

All pilots understand attitude, because this is determined by reference to the horizon. When that horizon is obscured or can't be seen at all and no surface references can help the pilot determine attitude, then attitude must be determined using instruments. Sounds straightforward, right? Well, most times it is, but occasionally, in low visibility for example, the pilots sense conflict with the information inside and outside the aircraft. In such an event, spatial disorientation can be said to have occurred [5]. Spatial disorientation comprises a number of illusions that can be broken down in the following categories:

1. Vestibular System
2. Visual/Night
3. Landing
4. Atmospheric

4.5.1 Vestibular System Illusions

This category of illusions is caused by sensory mismatches in the inner ear. It includes: The Leans, the Coriolis Illusion, the Graveyard Spin, the Graveyard Spiral, the Somatogravic Illusion and the Inversion Illusion. We'll cover each of these in a moment, but first we need to orient ourselves to the vestibular system (◘ Fig. 4.6).

We humans *sense* our position in three-dimensional space. Some of that sensory information is detected by *proprioceptors* in the muscles, tendons and joints. This information interacts with more sensory information generated by touch, pressure, hearing and—the vestibular system. All this sensory information is channeled to the brain, where it is processed to provide you with position and motion information. If you receive good information, then you can determine your body orientation and speed and maintain your balance. But if the brain receives limited or distorted sensory inputs, disorientation can occur. For example, sensory inputs received by the brain during the execution of high-G turns or spins are unusual inputs and can create compelling illusions that may cause a pilot to react dangerously. There is nothing wrong with the vestibular system in this case; it is just that it is a system that is not naturally adapted to flight.

4.5.2 Vestibular System Function and Anatomy

In a nutshell, the vestibular system makes sense of signals received from the vestibular receptors in the inner ear and stretch receptors in muscles to provide spatial orientation, gaze stability and maintain proper posture and balance. Before we look at how these signals may be disrupted to cause illusions, it is important to familiarise ourselves with the structure of the vestibular system.

Take a look at ◘ Fig. 4.7. As you can see, the inner ear comprises a hearing component (cochlea) and a balance component (vestibular apparatus). From a pilot's

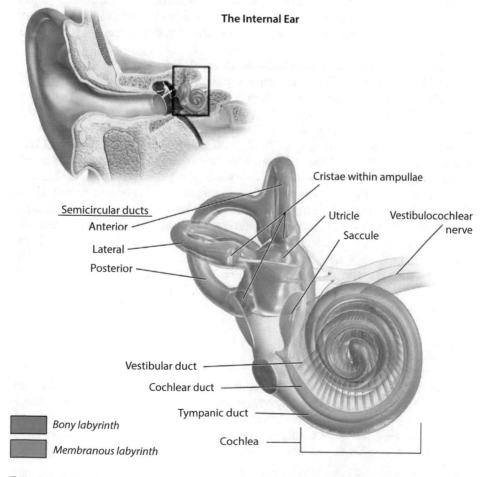

The Internal Ear

Cristae within ampullae

Semicircular ducts
Anterior
Lateral
Posterior

Utricle
Saccule

Vestibulocochlear nerve

Vestibular duct
Cochlear duct
Tympanic duct

Bony labyrinth

Membranous labyrinth

Cochlea

◘ Fig. 4.7   Internal ear anatomy. Credit: Blausen.com staff (2014). Medical gallery of Blausen Medical 2014

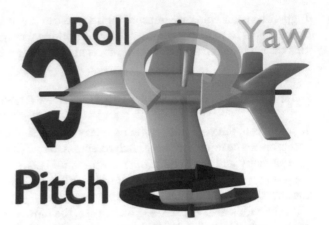

◘ Fig. 4.8   Pitch, roll and yaw in an aircraft. Credit: Zero One

perspective, we are particularly interested in those three semicircular canals and the utricle and saccule. That's because the semicircular canals are sensitive to angular accelerations of the head. The anterior, posterior and horizontal semicircular canals are arranged at 90° to one another, which means they can detect changes in pitch, roll and yaw (◘ Fig. 4.8).

That's great for knowing your orientation as a pilot, but what about speed and acceleration? Well, that's where the utricle and saccule come into play: these two parts—collectively called the *otolith organs*—of the vestibular system provide you with dynamic changes in linear motion and acceleration of your head, useful for when you're accelerating an aircraft on a runway. To do their job, the semicircular canals and the otolith organs rely on a specialized receptor cell known simply as the hair cell. Each of these hair cells, which are embedded in the semicircular canals and in the otolith organs in a gelatinous mass, contains more than 50 very small *cilia*. When you move, the hair cells and cilia move in the gelatinous mass and deflection of the cilia generates nerve signals. The problem with this arrangement is that the vestibular system can be tricked. Imagine you are in a turn, and as you turn the cilia are deflected, providing your brain with information that you are turning. So far so good, right? It sounds simple, but if you continue the turn, the system "catches up" and those cilia return to the vertical position, telling the brain that you are no longer turning. The impulse then is to tighten the turn, and before you know it you are in a *graveyard spiral*. Which brings us to the subject of vestibular system illusions.

4.5.3 Somatogyral Illusions

The Leans (◘ Fig. 4.9) can occur when a pilot makes a quick correction to a banked attitude that has been entered too slowly. When this happens, it is possible that the sensory information from your inner ear tells your brain that you are banking in the opposite direction. An experienced pilot will perform an instrument scan and roll the aircraft level. An inexperienced pilot may become so disoriented by this illusion that they may roll the

Fig. 4.9 The Leans.
Credit: boldmethod

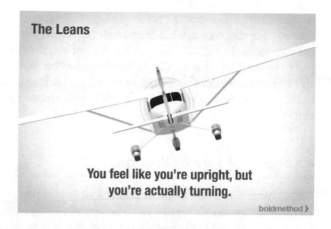

Fig. 4.9 The Leans.
Credit: boldmethod

Fig. 4.10 Graveyard spiral.
Credit: boldmethod

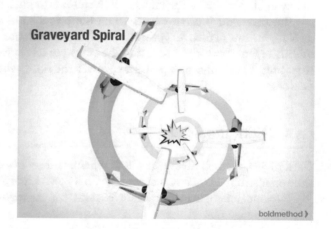

aircraft. The Leans is the most common visual illusion in flying. The most dangerous is the Coriolis Illusion. Both of these illusions, together with the Graveyard Spiral, are known as Somatogyral (from the word 'gyre' meaning spiral) Illusions.

The Coriolis Illusion occurs when a pilot is in a turn and bends their head downward or backward. A pilot may do this to check the chart or perhaps check an overhead panel. The problem is that either of these movements creates angular motion of the head that is different than the plane of the aircraft—while the pilot is turning, one of the semicircular canals is activated, but when the pilot looks up or down, another of the semicircular canals is activated. Simultaneous stimulation of two semicircular canals generates a compelling sensation that the aircraft is rolling, pitching *and* yawing. In addition to be compelling, such a situation can cause vertigo with the result that the pilot quickly becomes disoriented and loses control of the aircraft.

The Graveyard Spiral (**Fig. 4.10) is another turning illusion, in this case a tight, descending turn. To start, the pilot may begin a very gradual roll and not realize it. The

4

problem with this is that the vestibular system does not sense roll rates that are less than two degrees per second. So, as the aircraft begins to spiral downwards, the rate of descent increases and the pilot detects the descent but not the turn. Another scenario is when a pilot intentionally makes a turn, but because the bank angle is so gradual, the pilot thinks more and more control inputs must be made. And if these control inputs are less than two degrees per second, the result is a tightened turn and an eventual graveyard spiral.

4.5.4 Somatogravic Illusions

This class of illusion includes the Somatogravic and Inversion Illusions. The first one has its roots in the otolith organs. In an acceleration that occurs during takeoff, the otolith organs are stimulated to create the illusion of being nose-up. This sensation is amplified in low light conditions. The impulse of the pilot is to push the nose down.

The Inversion Illusion occurs when there is a sudden change from climbing to level flight. This maneuver generates excessive stimulation of linear acceleration in the otolith organs, with the result that the pilot perceives the aircraft to be inverted or tumbling. The common response is to lower the nose, which intensifies the illusion… or worse.

4.5.5 Night Illusions

Dark nights often eliminate the pilot's reference to the visual horizon, requiring a reliance on instruments, a task that comes with its own set of challenges, including illusions [6]. Pilots are taught to identify these illusions, but the night sky can be especially deceptive. And dangerous.

False Horizon   This illusion usually occurs on particularly dark nights when the pilot has no reference to a visual horizon. The pilot may search for the horizon and mistake a layer of clouds as the visual horizon. This can result in incorrect attitude inputs being made.

Autokinesis   This is caused by staring at a point of light against a dark background for several seconds. When a pilot does this, the light appears to move, causing the pilot to lose control of the aircraft while attempting to align it with the light.

Black Hole Illusion   Sometimes known as the Black Hole Approach, this illusion (◘ Fig. 4.11) occurs on approach over water or unlit terrain. Imagine you are preparing for landing at night and the only lights you can see are the runway lights. As you make your approach, you have no peripheral visual cues to help you land, which means you will have difficulty orienting yourself relative to the horizon. This set of circumstances means that the runway can appear out of position because it will be difficult to judge distance, especially if the pilot confuses the approach and runway lights.

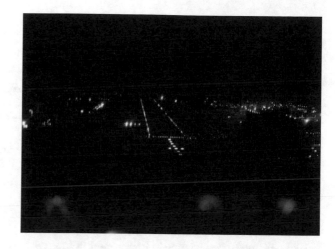

◘ Fig. 4.11 San Juan runway at night, San Juan, Puerto Rico. Credit: Jaro Nemčok

4.5.6 Landing Illusions

This category of illusions (Appendix V) is caused by atmospheric conditions and surface features such as runways.

Upsloping and Downsloping Runways These illusions are caused by either an upsloping or a downsloping runway. When the runway is upsloping, the pilot has the illusion that the aircraft is higher than it actually is. This type of illusion can lead to a *lower approach*. When the pilot is faced with a downsloping runway, he/she is faced with an illusion that the aircraft is lower than it is. This type of illusion can result in a *higher approach*.

Runway Width A runway that is narrower than usual can create the illusion that the aircraft is higher than it actually is, which may cause the pilot to fly an approach that is lower than normal. Conversely, a runway that is wider than usual may have the opposite effect, with the result that the pilot may overshoot the runway. Why might this happen? Imagine you're a student pilot who has been solely flying at a small airstrip that features a narrow runway. Then the day arrives for your first cross-country flight, and one of the airports you must visit features a runway that is five or six times wider than your home runway!

Atmospheric Illusions There are all sorts of meteorological phenomena that may cause pilots to become disoriented. For example: surface reference to the horizon may be obscured by smoke or fog; sunlight shining through clouds may affect vision; rain on the windscreen can cause water refraction, which can cause pilots to think they are higher than they actually are; and haze can cause pilots to perceive they are farther from the runway than they are. Conversely, extremely clear conditions can present the illusion of being closer to the runway, which may cause the pilot to overshoot as a result of a high approach [1].

4.5.7 Preventing Illusions

Illusions are commonplace in the aviation arena, and without a proper understanding of the various motions and forces that cause them, the pilot will be unprepared to take avoiding action. The steps pilots should take to prevent being a victim of one of these illusions are discussed here.

1. Visual reference must be made to reliable, fixed points on the ground or to flight instruments
2. Anticipation and planning are key. If you are flying to an unfamiliar airport, it is important to consult airport diagrams, runway slope, lighting and terrain
3. Use the Precision Approach Path Indicator or Visual Approach Slope Indicator for visual reference whenever these systems are available
4. Make frequent use of instruments, especially the altimeter during night flying
5. To reduce loss of spatial disorientation:
   (i) Maintain proficiency in instrument flying
   (ii) Maintain currency when flying at night
   (iii) Familiarize yourself with unique geographical conditions
   (iv) Check weather forecasts prior to departure
   (v) Rely on instruments unless the natural horizon is clearly visible

And what of Gosden, whom we mentioned at the beginning of this section? Well, he survived his mission thanks to his aircraft's forward-looking infrared (FLIR) system, which helped him identify a line of infrared lights that marked a column of American armored vehicles on the ground. Although he couldn't see the ground, the vehicles provided him with sufficient information to allow him to land safely. The FLIR system Gosden used helped him reduce the chances of him suffering from spatial disorientation at night. Under clear weather conditions the FLIR system works well, but its performance can be compromised by factors such as terrain contrast and dust particles.

4.6 Vision Issues and Medical Certification

While pilots usually have better vision than the general population, they are not immune to the effects of aging. As we get older, the risk of cataracts and glaucoma increase and the sharpness of our vision decreases [7, 8]. In some cases it might be possible to correct an age-related vision problem by surgery or by lens implants, but these procedures may affect medical certification, so it is useful to understand how some of the more common vision conditions may impact your ability to fly.

First, you may be surprised how many Americans are affected by visual impairment. According to the American Academy of Ophthalmology (AAO), the organization that tracks data on this sort of thing, 22 million Americans over the age of 40 are affected by cataracts, 2.3 million are affected by glaucoma, 150 million wear corrective eyewear, and 36 million wear contact lenses [9]. In addition to those stats, almost one million Americans undergo refractive surgical procedures every year. So, if you're reading this, there's a very good chance that you fit into one or more of those statistics. How does it affect your flight medical? Let's take a look.

4.6.1 Cataracts

Sometime after you turn 50, there is a chance your doctor will inform you that you have cataracts (◨ Fig. 4.12). Your first course of action will probably be to investigate the condition (Aside) before wondering how having cataracts will affect your flying [9].

Aside

Cataracts

A cataract is a clouding of the lens of the eye. As you age, the cloudiness in your lens becomes greater and greater, until eventually vision impairment is so severe that it is impossible to pass even the 3rd-class medical certificate. Unfortunately, cataracts is a condition that cannot be corrected by simply wearing glasses.

4.6.2 Cataract Surgery

One remedy for cataracts is to simply remove the cloudy lens and insert an artificial lens (known as an intraocular lens (IOL) in the field of ophthalmology) into the eye. The problem with this procedure is that it is not covered by most private insurance plans until distance vision is impaired to 20/50. For pilots there may be a way around this by submitting documentation stating that significant lifestyle changes—unemployment!— may result if corrective surgery is not performed. Pilots holding 1st class medical certificates should definitely explore this option. For those hesitant about surgery, there is not much to be concerned about; the surgery takes only 15 minutes, recovery time is about a month, and the result of the surgery is long-lasting clear vision. The surgeon will use a high-frequency ultrasound instrument that breaks up the cloudy lens into fragments that are removed by suction, a procedure called phacoemulsification. Once this is done, the surgeon simply inserts the IOL and carefully positions it behind your iris and pupil in the same place that your original lens occupied. A protective shield is then placed over your eye to secure the IOL in the early stages of cataract recovery.

◨ **Fig. 4.12** Cataracts. Credit: Rakesh Ahuja, MD

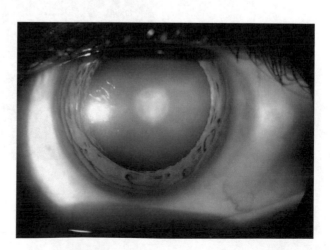

4.6.2.1 Laser-Assisted Cataract Surgery

Another procedure to correct cataracts is laser surgery, more commonly known as LASIK[1] (■ Fig. 4.13). This procedure, which is approved by the FDA, requires the surgeon to use a laser to create a corneal incision. The surgeon then removes the anterior capsule of the lens and fragments the cataract before creating peripheral corneal incisions to correct the vision impairment.

4.6.2.2 Preparing for Cataract Surgery

Before your surgery, your ophthalmologist will conduct an eye exam to determine your eye health and the extent of your nearsightedness, farsightedness and/or astigmatism. This exam will help the surgeon select the best IOL[2] to give you the best possible vision.

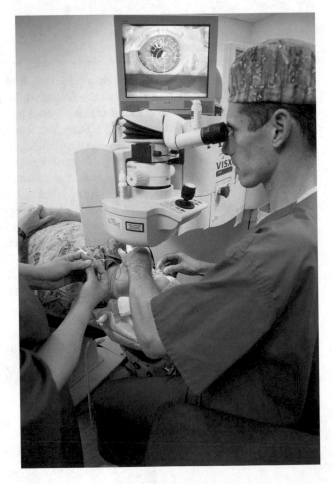

■ Fig. 4.13 Bethesda, Md. (May 1, 2007). Capt. Joseph Pasternak, an ophthalmology surgeon at National Naval Medical Center Bethesda, lines up the laser on Marine Corps Lt. Col. Lawrence Ryder's eye before beginning LASIK VISX surgery. The actual procedure can take only seconds. The new VISX procedure only takes days for service member's to recover, whereas the old PRK procedure took months. Credit: US Navy photo by Mass Communication Specialist 1st Class Brien Aho. USN

---

1   Laser in situ Keratomileusis is a procedure performed by blade-free IntraLase or Allegretto wave lasers
2   The FAA permits the use of FDA-approved IOLs for all classes of medical certification

On the day of the surgery, be prepared to be at the clinic for about 90 minutes and arrange for someone to drive you home! You will be given some eye drops to use several times a day for a few weeks following your surgery, and you can expect some blurriness and eye redness during this period.

Then, once your ophthalmologist has released you to resume normal activities, you can arrange for an eye exam with your aviation medical examiner—be sure to take along Report of Eye Evaluation (FAA Form 8500-7) with you. Provided you meet the visual acuity standards for the class of medical certificate you have applied for, you will be issued a medical certificate.

4.6.3 Other Eye Conditions

4.6.3.1 Myopia

If you have myopia, you will not be able to see distant objects clearly without corrective lenses. A pilot with this condition will probably see quite well during the day, but at night they will have difficulty seeing blue-green, and as light levels decrease the focusing mechanism of their eye may increase their myopia.

4.6.3.2 Hyperopia

Those with hyperopia have difficulty seeing objects up close but have no trouble seeing distant objects in sharp contrast.

4.6.3.3 Astigmatism

This condition is caused by an irregularly shaped cornea, which may cause objects to be viewed out of focus [8].

4.6.3.4 Presbyopia

This condition is a part of the aging process and is the deterioration of the ability of your eyes to focus on near objects. As the condition gets worse, you will find it increasingly difficult to read maps and checklists. Fortunately, like most these conditions, the problem can be corrected with a pair of adjusted glasses.

4.6.3.5 Glaucoma

This condition is one of the leading causes of vision impairment in adults aged 60 years and older. There are two types, Open-angle (chronic) Glaucoma and Closed-angle (acute) Glaucoma. In Open-angle Glaucoma, the buildup of fluid may take several months or even years. Closed-angle Glaucoma is less common but potentially more damaging, primarily because of the speed with which it strikes. Neither condition is curable or reversible, but once it is diagnosed it is possible to mitigate against further vision loss. If you are a pilot, the first step will be to complete Glaucoma Eye Evaluation Form 8500-14 and submit it to your AME.

4.6.3.6 Contact Lenses

If you wear single vision contacts you may resume flying immediately, providing you meet FAA vision standards [10]. If you wear color-tinted lenses you may only fly if the lenses do not significantly reduce light. For bifocal/multifocal lenses, you must have worn the lenses for at least one month to allow time for your eyes to adapt. You will also need to provide a FAA report of an eye evaluation to show you meet the vision standards for your class of medical certification.

4.7 Summary

4

The misperceptions, vision issues and illusions discussed in this chapter exist because the human vision system was not designed for flight. Sadly, in many instances, we have only learned about the limitations of our visual and perceptual systems through accidents. Unreliable environmental cues, overconfident pilots or a pilot's own preference for visual flying each conspire to bring about aviation incidents, and it is only through a thorough understanding of the limitations of the human visual system that such incidents can be avoided.

Key Terms
AAO - American Academy of Ophthalmology
FLIR - Forward-looking Infrared
FoV - Field of View
IOL - Intraocular Lens
LASIK - Laser in situ Keratomileusis
OCVT - Operational Color Vision Test
PAPI - Precision Approach Path Indicator
VASI - Visual Approach Slope Indicator

Review Questions
1. Explain what is meant by field of view
2. What is the difference between photopic, mesopic and scotopic vision?
3. Explain what is meant by the term vergence
4. List five factors that may affect vision
5. Explain the difference between somatogravic and somatogyral illusions
6. Describe how a pilot may experience the Leans
7. What illusions might be experienced by a pilot approaching an upsloping runway and wide runway?
8. What is the difference between hyperopia and presbyopia?
9. What is ocular pursuit?
10. What do the otolith organs do?

References

1. Hughes, P.K., Vingrys, A.J.: Reduced contrast sensitivity when viewing through an aircraft windscreen. Aviat. Space Environ. Med. **62**(3), 254–257 (1991)
2. Mertens, H.W.: Comparison of the visual perception of a runway model in pilots and non pilots during simulated night landing approaches. Aviat. Space Environ. Med. **49**(9), 1043–1055 (1978)
3. O'Brien, K.A., Cole, B.L., Maddocks, J.D., Forbes, A.B.: Color and defective color vision as factors in the conspicuity of signs and signals. Hum. Factors. **44**(4), 665–675 (2002)
4. Holmes, S.R., Bunting, A., Brown, D.L., Hiatt, K.L., Braithwaite, M.G., Harrigan, M.J.: Survey of spatial disorientation in military pilots and navigators. Aviat. Space Environ. Med. **74**(9), 957–965 (2003)
5. Braithwaite, M.G., Douglass, P.K., Durnford, S.J., Lucas, G.: The hazard of spatial disorientation during helicopter flight using night vision devices. Aviat. Space Environ. Med. **69**(11), 1038–1044 (1998)
6. DeVilbiss, C.A., Ercoline, W.R., Antonio, J.C.: Visual performance with night vision goggles (NVGs) measured in USAF aircrewmembers. In: Lewandowski, R.J., Stephens, W., Haworth, L.A. (eds.) SPIE Proceedings, Helmet and Helmet-Mounted Displays and Symbology Design Requirements, vol. 2218, pp. 64–70. SPIE-The International Society for Optical Engineering, Bellingham (1994)
7. Sekuler, A.B., Bennett, P.J., Mamelak, M.: Effects of aging on the useful field of view. Exp. Aging Res. **26**(2), 103–120 (2000)
8. Gudmundsdottir, E., Jonasson, F., Jonsson, V., Stefansson, E., Sasaki, H., Sasaki, K.: "With the rule" astigmatism is not the rule in the elderly. Reykjavik Eye Study: a population based study of refraction and visual acuity in citizens of Reykjavik 50 years and older. Iceland-Japan Co-Working Study Groups. Acta Ophthalmol. Scand. **78**(6), 642–646 (2000)
9. Brabyn, J.A., Haegerstroem-Portnoy, G., Schneck, M.E., Lott, L.A.: Visual impairments in elderly people under everyday viewing conditions. J. Vis. Impair. Blind. **94**(12), 741–755 (2000)
10. Bachman, W.G.: Evaluation of extended wear soft and rigid contact lens use by Army aviators. J. Am. Optom. Assoc. **61**(3), 203–210 (1990)

Suggested Reading by Topic
General Reference Material

Gibb, R., Gray, R., Scharff, L.: Aviation Visual Perception: Research, Misperception and Mishaps (Ashgate Studies In Human Factors for Flight Operations), 1st edn. Routledge, London/New York (2010)

General Articles Published by Aviation Agencies

https://www.faa.gov/other_visit/aviation_industry/designees_delegations/designee_types/ame/
https://www.faa.gov/tv/?mediaId=467
https://www.faa.gov/pilots/safety/pilotsafetybrochures/media/pilot_vision.pdf

Web References

http://webvision.med.utah.edu
http://www.handprint.com/HP/WCL/color1.html
http://www.psy.ed.ac.uk
http://web.mit.edu/bcs/schillerlab/research.html

Altitude and G-Forces

© Springer Nature Switzerland AG 2020
E. Seedhouse et al., *Human Factors in Air Transport*,
https://doi.org/10.1007/978-3-030-13848-6_5

Learning Objectives

After completing this chapter, you should be able to
- Describe hypoxia
- Explain why slow onset hypoxia is so dangerous
- Describe a rapid decompression
- Explain the difference between GOR and ROR
- Describe how a pilot might suffer from G-LOC
- Explain what is meant by hydrostatic pressure

5 5.1 Introduction

Several physiological problems can affect pilots during flight. One of the most danger-ous problems is *hypoxia*, defined as the lack of sufficient oxygen in the blood, cells and/or tissues to allow for continued normal physiological activity [1]. Hypoxia is prevented by maintaining a cabin altitude below 8,000 feet MSL. Flying above 10,000 feet MSL in a non-pressurized aircraft without supplemental oxygen, a malfunction of the pressur-ization system or oxygen system, or a rapid decompression can cause a deficiency of oxygen and will impair pilots if they do not recognize the effects on their bodies.

5.2 Slow Onset Hypoxia

Slow onset hypoxia is associated with malfunction or failure of an aircraft's pressurization system during climb or with a slow depressurization while at cruise altitude when dis-tracted by another emergency or technical problem. Whether by malfunction or an improperly positioned switch or setting on a pressurization management panel (which has happened, tragically), as the aircraft climbs, the cabin altitude continues to slowly climb past the planned cabin altitude. A slow leak around the seal of a door could also cause a very slow loss of pressure. Becoming fixated on the other issue, the crew might miss or silence the unexpected cabin altitude warning (aural or visual) that occurs as cabin altitude climbs past 10,000 feet MSL, and less and less oxygen to the brain eventually leads to incapacitation. Vision is the first sense to be affected, however hearing is somewhat resistant to hypoxia, and some crewmembers have been saved from disaster by directive radio calls from ATC or pilots of other aircraft, recognizing the signs in a pilot's voice.

This insidious form of hypoxia can be very difficult to identify when task-saturated in the cockpit. Pilots train in hypobaric chambers, or altitude chambers, to simulate the effects of high altitude on the human body. During training, pilots experience slow onset hypoxia (as well as rapid decompression, discussed in the next section) in a safe, controlled environment to familiarize themselves with their own symptoms. An observer will notice the pilot breathing more deeply, lips and nails becoming blue (cya-nosis), confusion or anger, poor judgment, possibly becoming euphoric, losing muscu-lar coordination, and eventually losing consciousness. Personal symptoms vary from person to person, and while many people will experience the same symptoms, they may appear in a different order and in varying intensities [1]. The pilot may notice signs such as nausea, headache, euphoria, dizziness, confusion, difficulty concentrating, loss of

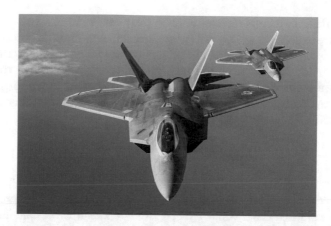

◘ Fig. 5.1 Although hypoxia cases are rare, the condition was highlighted in the media in 2010, after the loss of an F-22 Raptor and its pilot following a suspected oxygen loss. This incident highlighted physiological issues with the F-22, including a dozen hypoxia-like incidents between 2008 and 2011. For a time, the F-22 was grounded pending an investigation and resolution of the hypoxia issue. In 2012, following a House Armed Services Committee hearing it was found that the F-22 issues were not due to the supply of oxygen but a valve that controlled the pilot's pressure vest which could allow the vest to inflate unnecessarily, thereby restricting the pilot's ability to breathe. Credit: USAF

color vision, tunnel vision, blurred vision, tingling, numbness or fatigue. There may be other symptoms. In an altitude chamber, if the pilot does not correct the situation by putting on an oxygen mask after recognizing a few symptoms, the observer will put the mask on the pilot. The observer often puts the mask on for the pilot after directing the pilot to do so, finding the pilot unable to follow directions.

Of all the symptoms, headache and nausea are the only noticeably uncomfortable ones. Visual impairment is rarely noticeable and occurs slowly. A fixation on flying duties may keep the pilot so busy and distracted that the symptoms are not noticed. In an aircraft, with an entire crew suffering the effects together, judgment becomes extremely poor, and unless a controller detects the problem and can convince a member of the crew there's a problem, the crew is unlikely to recover. Luckily, recovery is rapid once 100% oxygen is administered in an altitude chamber, taking only a few seconds.

Hypoxia is a constant threat. Knowing one's symptoms and knowing the aircraft oxygen and pressurization systems are important to every pilot (◘ Fig. 5.1).

In 2005, a Boeing 737 operating as Helios Airways 522 crashed, killing everyone on board, as a result of the crew being overcome by hypoxia. The night prior to the accident, the aircraft had undergone maintenance and the pressurization system checked. The mode selector, always left in the "Auto" mode, had been left in the "Manual" mode inadvertently. Though pre-departure checklists should have caught the unusual switch position, the crew did not note the out-of-position switch. During climbout, passing through 10,000 feet, the cabin altitude alert warning sounded. The crew mistook the warning for an erroneous takeoff configuration warning as the sounds were identical, and then passing 14,000 feet, the passenger oxygen masks deployed along with a Master Caution light.

Additional issues caused the crew to contact Helios' maintenance base for advice as the aircraft continued to climb. Radio contact ended as the aircraft climbed through

5

28,900 feet. The crewmembers never donned their oxygen masks, believing the problems they were experiencing were not related to cabin pressure. The aircraft continued its climb to 34,000 feet, connected to the autopilot, and followed its programmed flight path until entering holding near Athens, Greece. Attempts to contact the crew were futile, and two F-16s were launched to intercept the aircraft. The F-16 pilots did not observe the captain but could see the first officer apparently unconscious and slumped over the controls. The aircraft eventually ran out of fuel and crashed [2].

5.3 Rapid Decompression

Structural failure of modern-day aircraft is uncommon, but metal fatigue or failure of a door seal or a cracked cabin window or pressure bulkhead is possible. Pilots practice rapid decompression and emergency descent procedures at least yearly in recurrent training, and while they can be approximated in a simulator, there's nothing like the rush of air, noise, fogging, flying debris and confusion that can accompany the real thing. An actual rapid decompression occurs within 1–10 seconds, often starting with a loud bang, usually accompanied by a blast of wind as the higher-pressure cabin air rushes out of the breach until cabin pressure equals the altitude outside the aircraft. Some have compared the sound to the popping of a cork, while others may not notice a sound at all, but the rush of air is unmistakable. Small, unsecured items may fly around as they get sucked into the stream of departing air. A fog will form, as the air in the cabin can carry much more moisture than the cold dry air outside and moisture condenses as the temperature and pressure drop [3]. The cabin temperature can fall to as low as −70°F to match the ambient temperature, depending on altitude. Confusion is common.

The speed with which cabin pressurization is lost also affects pilots' performance in recovery. The crew has only seconds to respond and take corrective action. Recognition, immediately donning oxygen masks and ensuring the positive flow of 100% oxygen, and rapidly descending to an altitude with breathable oxygen (usually 10,000 MSL) is the emergency procedure. Landing at the nearest suitable airfield where medical assistance is available is expected [1].

5.3.1 Time of Useful Consciousness

The Time of Useful Consciousness (TUC) is the period between a decompression or interruption of the supply of oxygen and the moment when the pilot is no longer able to take corrective action to protect him or herself (putting on an oxygen mask). The Effective Performance Time (EPT), often used interchangeably with TUC, is the time the pilot can effectively perform flying duties with inadequate oxygen [1]. ◘ Table 5.1 shows the TUC/EPT at various flight altitudes.

The above times assume a person at rest. Physical activity, stress, fatigue and a person's body condition will cause variation in times. Other factors include nutrition, alcohol and medication. A person with lower blood sugar is more prone to hypoxia, as is a person with alcohol in their system. Over-the-counter medication can cause cells not to use oxygen efficiently, thereby making the pilot less altitude resistant.

Table 5.1 TUC/EPT at various altitudes

ALTITUDE (feet MSL)	TUC/EPT
18,000	20–23 Min
22,000	10 Min
25,000	3–5 Min
28,000	2.5–3 Min
30,000	1–2 Min
35,0000	.5–1 Min
40,000	15–20 Sec
43,000	9–12 Sec
50,000	9–12 Sec

Adapted from ▶ FAA.gov [1], p. 3–3

5.3.2 Gravity and G-Forces

We are adapted to live and work in 1 G (gravity). And while we are on Earth, our body adapts very well to gravity because it is a constant force. But, when we pilot an aircraft, our experience of terrestrial G changes. This isn't surprising because by its very definition, flying an aircraft is all about overcoming gravity. The problem is that dealing with G in flight can cause serious problems for pilots who are unprepared. As you no doubt learned in school, the force of gravity causes a constant acceleration of 32 feet per second squared. So, an object falling to Earth will keep on accelerating at that speed until it reaches terminal velocity, which is the threshold at which the force of aerodynamic drag on the object overcomes the force or acceleration caused by G. This increase in acceleration is termed "Gs". A pilot entering a very steep turn can pull a lot of Gs. In some fighter aircraft such as the F-22 (**◘** Fig. 5.1), the Gs pulled can be in excess of 12. That's a real challenge for the body to deal with. As has been previously explained, aircraft operate along three axes, and because of this, Gs also act along these three axes (**◘** Fig. 5.2), which in turn leads to the categorization of G.

5.3.2.1 Categorization of G

There are three types of acceleration: Linear, Radial and Angular. Let's start with Linear.

- Linear Acceleration: This type of acceleration is simply the change of speed in a straight line. For example, when you are taking off or landing are experiencing linear acceleration.
- Radial Acceleration: This type of acceleration is experienced when you turn abruptly or if push over into a dive.
- Angular Acceleration: This type of acceleration is caused by a change of speed and direction. For example, when an aircraft spins, the pilot will be subjected to angular acceleration.

◻ **Fig. 5.2**   The G axes. Credit:
USAF/Aviation Medicine

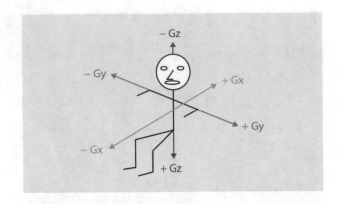

◻ **Fig. 5.3**   The centrifuge at
Wright-Patterson Air Force Base.
Credit: USAF

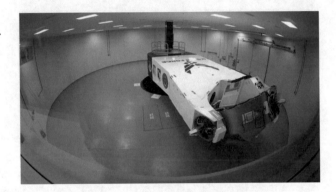

5.3.2.2 **G Forces**

The type and magnitude of G forces experienced by a pilot will depend on the flight control inputs. For example, in a takeoff roll, the predominant G force will be +Gx (from front to back), whereas when the pilot lands he/she will experience negative Gx or −Gx (from back to front). If the pilot decides to make a roll then he/she will experience lateral force, which is expressed as Gy. And the final G force is Gz. If this type of force is experienced from head to toe, it is termed positive Gz or +Gz, and if it is experienced from toe to head, it is termed negative Gz of −Gz (◻ Fig. 5.3).

5.3.2.3 **Physiological Effects of G**

As you can imagine, transitioning through these various types of G can cause havoc on the body. Imagine an aircraft beginning a pull-out from a steep dive. In this case the pilot will be loading his or her body with +Gz and the cardiovascular system must compensate. The job of the cardiovascular system is to keep blood flowing to the brain. Blood carries oxygen, and if the brain does not receive sufficient blood then the pilot will lose consciousness. This condition is termed gravity-induced loss of consciousness, or G-LOC.

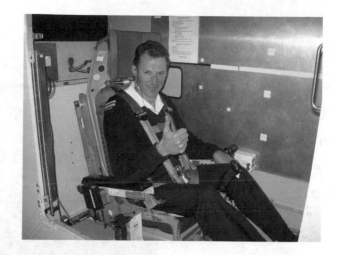

5.3.3 Signs and Symptoms of G

Going back to the pull-out example we just mentioned, the pilot will begin to suffer certain symptoms of increasing G as his or her cardiovascular system desperately tries to compensate. But the cardiovascular system can only do so much. As less and less blood reaches the brain, there is less oxygen reaching the eyes, with the result that peripheral vision begins to degrade. The pilot may suffer gray-out followed by black-out and ultimately G-LOC. G-LOC is deadly and has been the cause of several fatalities in aviation. When a pilot G-LOC's, they obviously lose control of the aircraft and the G's quickly subside, which means the pilot will begin to recover. But it generally takes about 15 seconds to recover consciousness and *another* 15 seconds to fully recover spatial awareness. That's 30 seconds! In 30 seconds, an aircraft can travel a fair distance.

How do we know so much about G? Pilots who want to fly high performance aircraft must be checked out in the centrifuge (☐ Fig. 5.4).

5.3.4 The Centrifuge

Before pilots sit in the centrifuge, they are taught some basic G physiology and then practice their anti G-straining maneuver (AGSM), which requires the pilots to take a deep breath in while simultaneously tensing the big muscles in the legs and abdomen, repeating the cycle every three seconds. The AGSM helps maintain hydrostatic pressure and ensures blood makes its way to the brain. To acquaint the pilots to G, the first run is at a gradual onset rate (GOR) of one tenth of 1 G per second. Once the pilot experiences their first symptom of G, which for most is a slight loss of peripheral vision, they begin their AGSM. This practice also provides the instructors an opportunity to evaluate the efficiency of the pilots' AGSM. Once the instructors are satisfied with the pilots' AGSM proficiency, the pilot will be prepared for a rapid onset rate (ROR) run, which will be at least 3 G per second. So, for example, a pilot who hopes to fly F-18's may have to perform a ROR

5

◘ Fig. 5.5 The author wearing
a G-suit, preparing for a high-G
flight in the BAe 146 Hawk.
Credit: Author

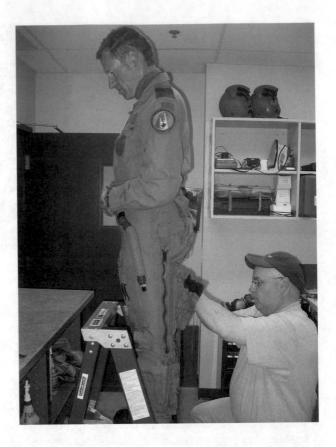

to 7 G while wearing an anti-G suit (◘ Fig. 5.5 - which provides between 1.6 and 2.2 G of protection). In an ROR run, the centrifuge accelerates from idling at 1.4 G to 7 G in less than 2 seconds, so the pilot must be prepared. Once at 7 G, the G's are held for 15 seconds so the pilot can demonstrate his or her AGSM to the instructors. It's quite a workout!

5.3.5 G Tolerance

While this training may seem straightforward, it is important for pilots to understand that G tolerance varies greatly from day to day. If you happen to fly aggressive G maneuvers daily, chances are that your body will become accustomed to G. But if you have to work at a desk for several months and you don't practice your AGSM, your body will lose that tolerance. This is why G-training is considered a perishable skill and why pilots must go through G training every 36 months in the military.

Time is not the only enemy of G tolerance. Alcohol, fatigue and dehydration will all conspire to increase susceptibility to G. Why does being dehydrated affect G tolerance? It's simple: your blood comprises 55% plasma, and plasma comprises 90% water, so your blood is effectively 50% water. Thus, if you become dehydrated, you lose blood volume and your body has to work extra hard to push sufficient blood to the head to prevent G-LOC.

Fatigue is another enemy. Pulling G is punishing and exhausting, so lack of physical conditioning will have a significant negative impact on a pilots ability to tolerate G.

5.3.6 G-Suits

Now you may think that the problem of G can be solved by wearing a G suit. Not so. The G suit, depending on the manufacturer, will provide between 1.6 and 2.2 G (Libelle suit for example) of protection. An AGSM performed effectively will provide about 3 G of protection. The G suit comprises an ensemble of tight-fitting trousers that can be fitted under or over the flight suit. Integrated into the trousers is a system of bladders that pressurize when high G is detected (the G suit is plugged into the aircraft). The pressurization of the bladders exerts pressure on the legs and the abdomen, ensuring that blood doesn't drain away from the brain.

5.4 Summary

In this chapter we discussed the physiological problems that may affect pilots during flight. Of these problems, the most dangerous is *hypoxia*. Hypoxia is prevented by maintaining cabin altitude, but a malfunction of the aircraft's pressurization system and/or oxygen system may result in slow onset hypoxia or a rapid decompression. If this happens, it is important that pilots recognize the signs and symptoms and be able to act accordingly. We also discussed the effects of G. While this is not normally a challenge in general aviation, for those engaged in military aviation, the effects of G may be significant. And, like hypoxia, it is important that pilots understand the effects of the onset of G and be able to react effectively.

Key Terms
CRM - Crew Resource Management
EPT - Effective Performance Time
FAR - Federal Aviation Regulations
MSL - Mean Sea Level
TUC - Time of Useful Consciousness

Review Questions
1. What is hypoxia?
2. Why is slow onset hypoxia described as insidious?
3. What might cause slow onset hypoxia?
4. What caused the crew of Helios 522 to become hypoxic?
5. Describe a rapid decompression
6. What is Time of Useful Consciousness?

References

1. Federal Aviation Administration [FAA]: Introduction to aviation physiology. Retrieved from https://www.faa.gov/pilots/training/airman_education/media/IntroAviationPhys.pdf (n.d.)
2. Air Accident Investigation & Aviation Safety Board (AAIASB): Aircraft accident report: Helios Airways Flight HCY522 Boeing 737-31S at Grammatiko, Hellas on 14 August 2005. Retrieved from https://reports.aviation-safety.net/2005/20050814-0_B733_5B-DBY.pdf (2006, Nov)
3. Pendleton, L.D.: When humans fly high: What pilots should know about high-altitude physiology, hypoxia, and rapid decompression. Retrieved from AVweb website: https://www.avweb.com/news/aeromed/181893-1.html (1999, Nov 7)

Suggested Reading

5

Pendleton, L.D.: When humans fly high: What pilots should know about high-altitude physiology, hypoxia, and rapid decompression. Retrieved from the AVweb website: https://www.avweb.com/news/aeromed/181893-1.html (1999, Nov 7)

Pulling, G., Seedhouse, E.: Published by Springer-Praxis, 2012. ISBN-13: 978-1461430292

Information Processing

© Springer Nature Switzerland AG 2020
E. Seedhouse et al., *Human Factors in Air Transport*,
https://doi.org/10.1007/978-3-030-13848-6_6

Learning Objectives

After completing this section, you should be able to:

— Describe the factors affecting information processing
— Explain what is meant by situational awareness
— Describe the function of working memory
— Identify and describe the different sensory organs within the inner ear
— Explain the configuration and the purpose of the Semicircular canals
— Explain the purpose of the Otolith organs
— Describe how the movement of the Endolymph fluid effects the sensation of pitch, roll and yaw
— Identify the conflicts between the vestibular system and initial movement of the aircraft
— Describe the Vestibular and Somatosensory illusions and identify the correct responses
— Identify the best method to avoid Spatial disorientation

6.1 Introduction

Those employed in the aviation industry, whether they be pilots, controllers or maintenance workers, must process a myriad of information from a myriad of sources. They must be able to not only process this information but to also prioritize it, make decisions and take action. This process is termed *information processing*, and it essentially describes the ability of the human-in-the-loop to process information within a timeframe in a manner that ultimately leads to responses required for the task in hand.

6.1.1 Information Processing Capability

Information processing capability (◘ Fig. 6.1) varies greatly. It can be affected by the time of day, the environment and the task. It can also be affected by age, health, workplace, experience, distractions, stress and fatigue. Since there are so many variables that can affect our information processing capabilities, it is important to understand exactly how this human factor can be limited and how decision-making capabilities can be affected. Why? So that mistakes can be reduced. Common mistakes caused by reduced information processing include:

— Misunderstanding information
— Forgetting information
— Processing information incorrectly
— Recalling information incorrectly
— Reacting incorrectly

6.1.2 Situational Awareness and Information Processing

A key element in information processing is situational awareness (SA). What is SA? A basic definition can be found in work by Dominguez [1], who stated that SA (◘ Fig. 6.2) must include the following four elements:

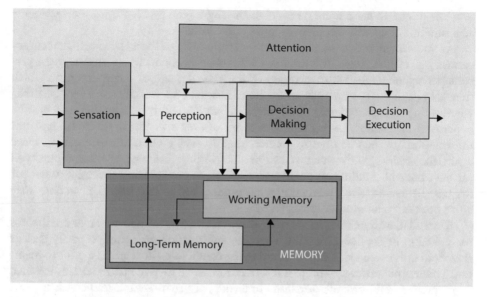

■ **Fig. 6.1**   Information processing model. Credit: FAA

■ **Fig. 6.2**   Situational awareness.
Credit: FAA

Situational Awareness (SA)

- The accurate perception and understanding of all the factors and conditions within the four fundamental risk elements that affect safety before, during, and after the flight (FAA-H-8083-25)

- Four Risk Elements:
  - Pilot
  - Airplane
  - enVironment
  - External pressures

1. Extracting information from the environment
2. Integrating this information with relevant internal knowledge to create a mental picture of the current situation
3. Using this picture to direct further perceptual exploration in a continual perceptual cycle
4. Anticipating future events

Based on the above definition, we know SA is based on our perception of the environment around us, and that perception is in turn based on sensory information. For example, information available to a pilot in the cockpit includes the primary flight display, engine instrument readouts, voice communication, data-links, vision and navigation data. But this isn't the only information the pilot relies on to build

SA. The pilot also has a mental model of the flight plan that includes such elements as a timeline of events, weather en-route and traffic.

As you can appreciate by now, SA is determined by so many factors that accuracy can vary greatly. That said, this accuracy is ultimately dependent on what degree a person's perception aligns with the reality of the situation and/or environment in which they are operating. For example, in familiar situations, SA is likely to be very accurate, whereas in a complex and/or novel environment SA will be less so. SA may also be dependent on memory, as we retain memory of events that have occurred, and this information can then be used to predict what SA may be in a future situation. Once again, the accuracy with which we can predict SA is determined by the complexity of the environment. Additionally, while we may able to predict fairly accurately what our SA may be for ourselves, predicting what others may do and how their actions may affect our SA is a lot more complex [2, 3].

Since all these dynamic factors conspire to affect SA, it is important that continuous mental effort be applied, especially when our information processing capacity is at its threshold or is exceeded. Under normal flying conditions, SA requires a pilot to maintain a mental picture of the complex interrelationship of myriad factors such as weather, configuration of the aircraft, proximity to terrain, obstructions and traffic. A loss of SA concerning one or more of these may result in dire consequences, such as controlled flight into terrain, loss of control or airspace infringement. On the flip side, SA may be compromised by external factors such as severe air turbulence, heavy icing or strong head winds. To maintain SA, the pilot's job is to sustain the mental picture he or she has of the flight situation, anticipating the potential for unexpected events and being able to respond appropriately. But how, exactly?

6.1.3 Stages of Information Processing

There are four stages in information processing: sensing, perceiving, decision making and motor action, as outlined in ◘ Fig. 6.3. In addition to these stages, information processing includes five elements of memory: sensory, working, short term, long term and motor skills. Each of these types of memory can be best thought of as a distinct function that supports our ability to create a mental model of the world [4].

6.2 Factors Affecting Information Processing

6.2.1 Vigilance

Vigilance describes our state of awareness, and it can range from high to low. Our state of vigilance can be enhanced or reduced depending on the environment. For example, during periods of boredom or fatigue, our state of vigilance will be subdued. This is important because our state of vigilance will positively or negatively affect our SA. On a flight-deck pilots must constantly remain vigilant of myriad data, including information from engine systems, communication, and external events such as traffic and weather.

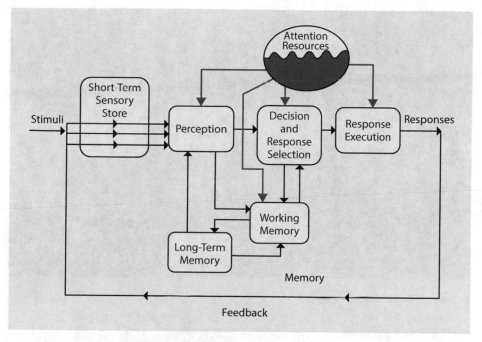

◘ Fig. 6.3 Factors affecting information processing. Credit: FAA

Of course, it is impossible to maintain a high state of vigilance *and* make sense of all this information, which is why pilots must pay attention to the most important data at any particular moment.

6.2.2 **Attention**

In addition to playing a role in our state of vigilance, attention is one of the determinants in our ability to multi-task, which in itself is an element of our information processing capability. There are a number of theories that explain how proficient we can be at multi-tasking, and they tend to agree on a number of determinant variables. For example, those of us who can divide attention between stimuli tend to be better multi-taskers than those that cannot do this. Multi-tasking is also affected by the intricacy or familiarity of the task—those tasks that are intricate demand our full attention, as do unfamiliar tasks. This is important because when we are attending completely to a task it means our vigilance is diluted, which in turn means we cannot turn our attention to any other task. Another aspect of attention is the degree to which our attention can be focused. For example, it is possible to be so absorbed in a task that we fail to hear the phone ring. In the world of aviation, pilots may so engrossed by, say, a night-time precision approach (◘ Fig. 6.4), that they fail to adjust their navigation aids. To prevent this from occurring, the design component of human factors comes into play, and consoles are designed to utilize visual and aural alarms to maintain attention.

6

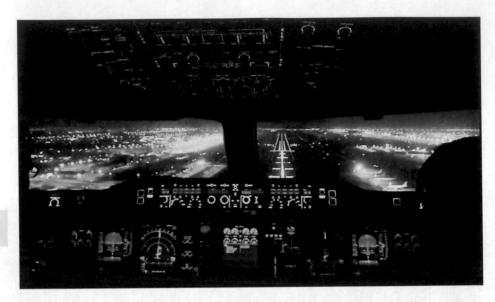

Fig. 6.4   Night landing. Credit: FAA

Fig. 6.5   Being aware of all sensory inputs. Credit: FAA

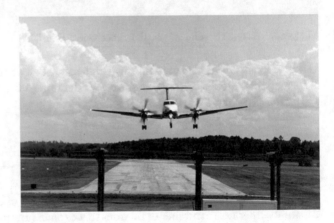

6.2.3 **Sensing**

A key element of information processing is *sensing*. Sensory inputs include *sound, light, pressure, taste* and *smell*. What is especially important in the context of information processing is that each of our senses has different sensory memories. For example, our visual memory lasts for less than one second, whereas our audible memory may last up to 8 seconds. As a pilot it is extremely important to pay attention to *all* sensory inputs (**Fig. 6.5**) in order to form a perception of the environment and thereby transfer sensory data into a more lasting memory [5]. Of course, all this takes effort and requires that the pilot engage their decision-making mechanism to help process all the information. One way that sensory inputs may be affected is by a deficiency in any one or more of our senses. For example, if our eyesight is not sharp, then visual inputs will not be processed very effectively. Equally, if our hearing is damaged then our ability to process aural inputs will be affected.

6.2.4 **Perception**

What do we do with all that sensory information? Well, we *process* it, which means *converting* that sensory information into something meaningful. We create an internal mental model or framework of the environment to the best of our ability. This model will always be a little rough around the edges, because it is impossible to collect and process all the data in the environment. But we can compensate for this, with one way being to use sensory information from past experiences to help smooth out those rough edges and create a more realistic model that is more in line with our expectations. An example? Think of a badly pixilated image of a famous face. Even though the image may be of low resolution, our brain can fill in the gaps and connect the dots so to speak. It is precisely this mechanism that allows us to divide attention and thereby multi-task.

Simple, right? Well, not quite. This mechanism, which helps us to multi-task, can be a double-edged sword that leads to misperception. The more you rely on past experiences, the more your expectations will alter your perception. Imagine a Canadian helicopter pilot who routinely flies along the pristine snow-covered forested valleys that are found pretty much anywhere in British Columbia. Over the years this pilot will have created a mental model of the trees being 50 meters tall. But, if he one day flies into a valley full of newly planted trees, he may fly closer to the ground than intended because he will have misperceived the scale. As you can imagine, such a scenario could have dire consequences, which is why it is so important to check and cross-check our perceptions with other inputs such as the altimeter and radar.

6.2.5 **Working Memory**

This type of memory, which is the memory that we use almost constantly to perform tasks, stores small amounts of data for short periods of time [6]. It is memory that is immediately accessible. An example of working memory in action is the pilot reading back an instruction from ATC. Once that task is complete, the information is usually lost within 30 seconds and replaced with new data and/or instructions. The limit of our working memory is between *5 and 7 pieces of information*, but this can be increased a little by *chunking*. For example, the telephone number 0014056374788 can be more easily remembered if is broken down into four chunks—001 405 637 4788. Another trick is to use mnemonics. Gradually, certain data/data-sets enter the long-term memory simply through repetition.

6.2.6 **Long-Term Memory**

As information is stored in our long-term memory it becomes more accessible, which means it becomes easier to recall when required. This is achieved through constant repetition of a task until it is almost automatic [6]. This works well for those tasks that are performed on a continuous basis, such as takeoffs and landings, but not so well for those tasks that are performed only intermittently or rarely, such as responding to an engine fire. This is why it is so important to at least practice rarely performed tasks to guard against loss of proficiency. One way to better understand how long-term memory works is to outline the manner in which data is stored. For long-term memory, data can be stored as semantic memory, episodic memory or unconsciously.

1. Semantic Memory. This memory category is our database. It contains facts and figures and is created by repetition and familiarity. It is this type of memory that helps us follow checklists and comply with instructions. One important point to note regarding semantic memory is that not everything that is stored there is correct. For example, if you are taught a checklist incorrectly, then you will remember it incorrectly. A second important point is that just because we have all these facts and figures stored in our semantic memory does not mean we can recall them instantly whenever necessary. This is because data that is rarely used becomes increasingly inaccessible with time and lack of practice.

2. Episodic Memory. This category of memory stores all our experiences and knowledge of events. As with all types of memory, the more often you recall a memory the easier it becomes to access that memory or experience. As you can appreciate, the recall of experiences can change with time, and recall will not always be immediate and identical.

3. Motor-Skills Memory. As we become more and more proficient in performing a task, we eventually attain a state when we can perform that task automatically and with almost no conscious effort. To understand how this occurs it is necessary to understand how learning a skill occurs. This can be broken down into the following four steps:

    (a) Unconscious incompetence
    (b) Conscious incompetence
    (c) Conscious competence
    (d) Unconscious competence

    As you can see from the sequence of phases, as we practice a skill it becomes increasingly less demanding until the fourth stage is reached, which is when the skill can be considered second nature. In fact, at this stage, the performance of the skill is so automated that we can free up information processing bandwidth to perform another task simultaneously. In other words, we are *multi-tasking*. Another way of thinking about this is to imagine our minds running different motor programs, and within each motor program there are several sub-programs, each kicking in when the situation demands.

6.2.7 **Deciding and Acting**

Deciding implies judgment, and in the world of aviation there are myriad skills that require this ability, for example judging when to communicate, when to solve problems and when to implement certain procedures. *Deciding* is all about decision making, and this is an acquired skill borne of knowledge and experience. In the context of information processing, the moment when we decide to do something is driven by selecting a particular action that best aligns with the task that must be performed. These actions can be either *skill-based*, *rule-based*, or *knowledge-based*. If you go back to the information processing model for a moment, you can see that when we decide to act, it is a decision driven by making corrections with the environment so we can perceive progress in the right direction. It is essentially an error-correcting, closed feedback loop [4]. Under most circumstances the process of making decisions works well, but when this decision-making process is accelerated and decisions must be made under pressure, it is more likely that accuracy may suffer and bad decisions may be made. It is under these circumstances that pilots increase their SA so they can react—by making the correct decision—appropriately.

6.2.8 Multi-Tasking

This skill is all about resource management, and there are some people who can manage this very well. Conversely, there are others who just don't have the aptitude for multi-tasking (◨ Fig. 6.6). But eventually, even the best of the best multi-taskers can only do so much [7]. If a person is given too many tasks, they ultimately reach the limit of their information processing capacity. When this happens, it is necessary to dump certain tasks, because if this not done, saturation occurs and performance takes a nosedive. To prevent this from happening, pilots utilize their crew resource management skills and delegate tasks as appropriate.

So, we've covered the key elements of information processing from a psychological perspective. Yet information processing is also determined by physiological mechanisms, specifically those housed in the vestibular system. This is where we turn our attention to in the next section.

6.2.9 Vertigo and Spatial Disorientation

As children, many of us played games where we intentionally induced dizziness, or the more clinically known term "vertigo". It may have started off when we were young with spinning around in circles, then watching one another attempt to walk a straight line or even simply maintain balance while standing. As we grew into our teenage years, we likely attended fairs for dizzying rides such as the roller coaster, tilt-a-whirl and other spinning amusements.

◨ **Fig. 6.6** USAF and IAF airmen work inside the cockpit of an IAF Ilyushin Il-76. Credit: Public domain

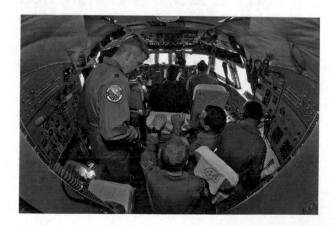

Imagine the same feelings and sensations affecting a pilot while flying an aircraft. This type of vertigo on the ground can be quite funny and enjoyable, yet to a pilot in the air, it can become extremely dangerous and life threatening.

In this section we will explore what is occurring inside your body and affecting your sense of balance, and how that relates to what you are observing with your eyes. You will learn why some pilots are affected and others are able to recognize the symptoms and take corrective action to prevent an accident. Why? How can other pilots protect themselves from experiencing vertigo?

Additionally, this section will discuss several actions that if taken will exacerbate the sensation of vertigo. Both the medical and physiological reasons contributing to this sensation will be explained. We will identify five specific times in flight when vertigo may become a problem and discuss the actions one can take to overcome or mitigate it. The procedures discussed in this section can help a pilot to identify the cause of vertigo and dizziness and then apply the correct methodology and procedures to overcome those feelings.

What is the definition of vertigo? A sensation of spinning or whirling motion that imparts a feeling of rotation of the subject or of objects around the subject in any plane. Vertigo is often used as a general term to describe dizziness (*Stedman's Medical Dictionary*, 28th Edition). Most of these symptoms originate within the Vestibular System, the sensory nerve pathways or the brain. Vertigo may be temporary or long term. Healthy bodies will normally resolve the sensation of vertigo without treatment, but underlying problems may require medical attention to overcome. The danger to pilots is that vertigo may induce Nystagmus, an uncontrolled eye movement that is usually an indication of a dysfunction of the inner ear or sensory pathways.

6.2.9.1 The Vestibular System

Several sensory systems help us to perceive how our body is positioned while operating in all types of environments. Whether it is walking, riding in an elevator, swimming, diving or flying an airplane, our sensory systems help us maintain a sense of balance and body position awareness. The senses of touch, vision and hearing work with the vestibular system to help prevent spatial disorientation. The vestibular system allows the pilot to sense movement and determine orientation in the surrounding environment. The main organs of the Vestibular system are located within the inner ear on each side of the human head and are about the size of a pea. The vestibular system is part of our sensory system and is responsible for detecting the movement and position of our head. The vestibular system (◘ Fig. 6.7a, b) also helps us to maintain our balance in all body positions and activities [8].

The vestibular system has three main organs: the semicircular canals, the otolith organs and the cochlea. The cochlea converts acoustic energy into neural information, which is sent to the brain and is used for processing auditory information. This discussion will cover the semicircular canals and the otolith organs. These are receptor organs responsible for detecting different types of linear and angular movement by monitoring the position and movement of the head. They work together to help maintain balance and equilibrium. The semicircular canals (◘ Fig. 6.8) are composed of three semicircular tubes filled with fluid, and they are positioned 90° apart from one another [9].

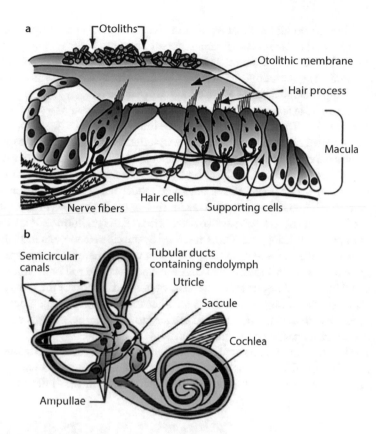

Fig. 6.7 The vestibular system showing the hair cells that are deflected during acceleration **a**, and the semicircular canals that detect angular acceleration **b**. Credit: USAF

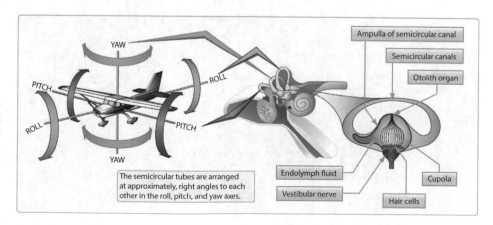

Fig. 6.8 The semicircular canals detect movement in pitch, roll and yaw. Credit: ▶ www. flightliteracy.com

The semicircular canals are filled with a fluid known as the endolymph fluid, which moves throughout the canal. These canals detect rotational movements of the head equating to pitch, roll and yaw, similar to a gyroscope. As the head moves about, the endolymph fluid moves through the canals. Within the canals is located a swelling known as the ampullae. Refer to ◘ Fig. 6.9.

Within the ampullae is embedded the cupula. Within the cupula is a series of receptor cells known as the cilia. The cilia receptors resemble fine vertical hairs, the purpose of which is to detect movement of endolymph fluid. The movement of the fluid in the canals causes these hair cells to bend and transmit a nerve impulse along the vestibular nerves to the brain. These impulses are sent as a result of each and every movement of the head in any plane. Rotating your head up or down affects the canal associated with pitch on an airplane. Rotating your head left to right affects the canal associated with yaw, and finally, tilting your head to the left or right affects the canal associated with roll. A condition to be aware of is the "lagging" or opposite direction of movement sensed by the cilia whenever a head movement in any direction is made. Newton's third law, "For every action, there is an equal and opposite reaction" governs this effect. When a pilot begins a climb, starts a roll or even yaws the aircraft, the endolymph fluid begins to move in the opposite direction of the movement. The fluid will then reverse and move in the correct direction shortly thereafter, but it initially gives a false sense of direction. This sensation can lead to incorrect action by the pilot, which will be discussed in the section on vestibular illusions (◘ Fig. 6.10).

The otolith organs are also located in the inner ear and are called the utricle and the saccule. These organs detect both vertical and horizontal movement such as going up and down in an elevator or acceleration and deceleration in a linear direction. Just as the

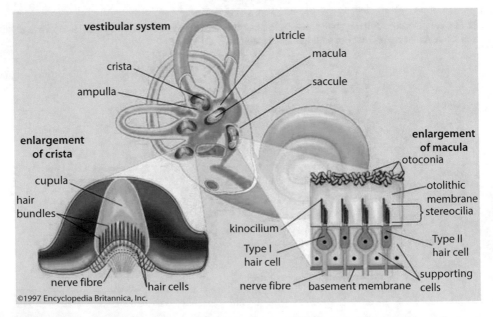

◘ **Fig. 6.9** The Neurovestibular system is designed to provide information about angular and linear acceleration thanks to the co-location of the semicircular canals and the otolith organs. Credit: *Encyclopedia Britannica*

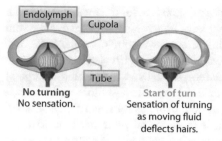

No turning
No sensation.

Start of turn
Sensation of turning
as moving fluid
deflects hairs.

Constant rate turn
No sensation after
fluid accelerates to
same speed as
tube wall.

Turn stopped
Sensation of turning in
opposite direction as
moving fluid deflects hairs
in opposite direction.

◻ **Fig. 6.10** The effect of rotation on the cilia in the neurovestibular system can provoke various aviation illusions. Credit: *Academy of Aeronautics and Aviation Sciences*

semicircular canals imitate a gyroscope, so these otolith organs simulate an instrument known as an accelerometer. The otolith organs are also filled with fluid similar to the endolymph fluid in the semicircular canals. Both organs contain small hair cells, cilia, projecting into the fluid contained within the organ.

Aside

The following are exercises to demonstrate the movement of the endolymph fluid within the Semicircular and Otolith organs.

Take a raw egg, lie it on its side an attempt to spin it. Initially, it will be hard to start the spinning as the yolk inside resists the forward motion. Thus, while the outer shell is moving in one direction, the inside yolk initially appears to move in the opposite direction. However, once the raw

egg begins to spin, if you quickly stop the shell and immediately release, the egg will start to spin again. This is because the fluid in the egg, the yoke, continues to move around for a short period.

Using the child's game of spinning around a bat, an individual can experience the effect of the endolymph fluid moving within the Semicircular canals as they drop the bat and try to walk or run in one direction.

Vertical and linear acceleration are experienced every day in our normal life. Quick starts in a car as well as fast stops affect the otolith organs. You experience a rearward force with acceleration and a forward force in a linear direction. However, with the otolith organs, once the fluid equalizes you cannot detect movement. When riding in an aircraft or automobile you detect the initial movement, but once the acceleration has stopped you have no idea of the speed. The otolith organs also detect vertical acceleration and deceleration. Riding in an elevator, you detect the initial vertical movement as the elevator begins to rise. You also detect the slowing down of the elevator as it begins to reach your desired floor. Once in motion, the fluid in the organs no longer moves and thus the cilia in the cupola do not detect movement; therefore, your sense of vertical or gravitational movement is not apparent. In much the same way, the otolith organs detect the initial acceleration when stepping onto a moving sidewalk. However, once walking on the moving sidewalk, the increased speed is not recognized until the sudden deceleration when stepping off the moving sidewalk.

The vestibular system is associated with the visual centers of the brain and influences the movement of a pilot's eyes. For example, when you tilt your head in any direction, the

Otolith organs along with the semicircular canals are responsible for the movement of your eyes keeping the eyes stable on where they were focused. Often these senses are moving your eyes opposite the movement of your head tilt. This is known as Vestibulo-Ocular Reflex and may be viewed on YouTube here (▶ https://www.youtube.com/watch?v=j_R0LcPnZ_w).

As we age, we progressively lose part of our receptor cells in the vestibular organs. For this reason, diminished balance and posture control affect seniors and increase their loss of balance. The vestibular system is quite reliable as long as there is a visual reference to the horizon or ground. However, if these visual references are lost, the vestibular system becomes unreliable. In this situation we have conflicting senses of vestibular versus ocular, which cause convincing illusions and bring about a dangerous condition known as vertigo or spatial disorientation. In this next section, we will discuss several common vestibular illusions (note: some of these illusions have been covered in ▶ Chapter 4, so what follows is a review). It is important that a pilot recognize the onset of this condition through training and awareness to reduce the chance of spatial disorientation.

6.2.9.2 Vestibular Illusions Attributed to the Semicircular Canals

Illusions involve both the semicircular canals and the somatogyral organs (utricle and saccula) of the vestibular system. These illusions usually occur when there is a loss of visual references, which may result in a false sense of rotation. Sometimes referred to as false illusions, the most common ones are discussed below.

Graveyard spiral and Graveyard spin   The graveyard spiral illusion may occur when a pilot enters a prolonged, constant rate turn. As this turn continues, the pilot may experience the illusion of not turning because the endolymph fluid and one of the semicircular canals has stabilized. Thus, the pilot has no sensation of a turn, but upon stopping the turn the fluid moves in the opposite direction, giving the pilot the erroneous sensation of turning in the opposite direction. The absence of the sensation of turning and the overcorrection and turn in the opposite direction will tighten the turn, possibly becoming a graveyard spin (◘ Fig. 6.11 and Appendix V).

The Leans   The most common vestibular illusion, which occurs when a pilot has experienced a prolonged, slight turn unnoticed. A pilot may be unaware of this slight turn, as a rotational direction of 2° per second or lower is below the threshold of the semicircular canals. The fluid in the canal will not rotate at this low rate of a turn and thus no indication is given to the pilot by the vestibular system. When the pilot notices the aircraft has turned and is off course, the pilot will roll wings level in order to stop the turn, sometimes resulting in the semicircular canals indicating a turn in the opposite direction even though the aircraft wings are now level. Thinking that the aircraft is banking in the opposite direction, a pilot may lean in the direction of the original turn or even roll in that direction attempting to perceive level flight. This is simply trying to overcome the vestibular perception of correct posture, resulting in a lean in the cockpit (◘ Fig. 6.12).

Coriolis illusion   Often known as the most deadly illusion. This occurs when there is simultaneous stimulation of two semicircular canals accompanied by the movement of the head in a different plane. It results from a turn and a tilting of the pilot's head in the turn. This solution usually occurs when a pilot is in a turn and looking down at an approach

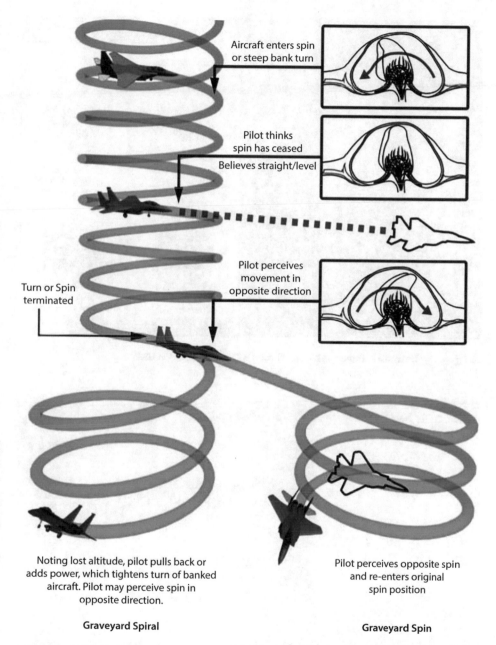

Aircraft enters spin
or steep bank turn

Pilot thinks
spin has ceased
Believes straight/level

Pilot perceives
movement in
opposite direction

Turn or Spin
terminated

Noting lost altitude, pilot pulls back or
adds power, which tightens turn of banked
aircraft. Pilot may perceive spin in
opposite direction.

Graveyard Spiral

Pilot perceives opposite spin
and re-enters original
spin position

Graveyard Spin

🔲 **Fig. 6.11**   The mechanism of the graveyard spiral. Credit: USAF

chart, map or other object. It will also occur in a turn with a pilot looking upward. The stimulation of these two semicircular canals will cause the pilot to become somewhat disoriented and perceive the aircraft is rolling pitching or turning in an unusual attitude. Often this will cause the pilot to maneuver the aircraft into a dangerous attitude and results in loss of control. For this reason, pilots should minimize head movement when banking, climbing or descending.

6

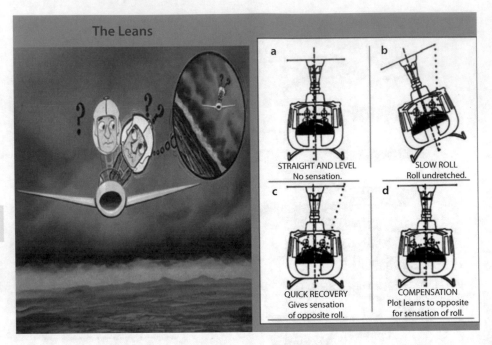

☐ Fig. 6.12 The most common vestibular illusion is "The Leans". Credit USAF

☐ Fig. 6.13 The inversion illusion. Credit: boldmethod

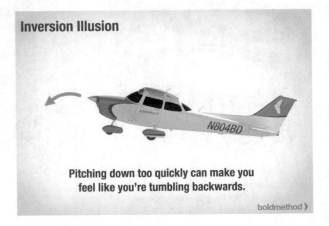

6.2.9.3 Vestibular Illusions Attributed to the Otolith Organs

The Inversion illusion   This illusion occurs when there is an abrupt change from a climb to straight and level flight. This movement stimulates the otolith organs, creating a sense of vertical movement that results in a sensory perception/illusion that the aircraft is inverted or tumbling backwards. Often, the pilot, having sensed the upward movement, may abruptly pushed the nose down, which simply exacerbates the feeling of vertical upward movement (☐ Fig. 6.13).

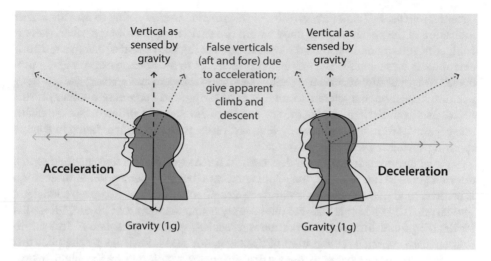

◻ Fig. 6.14 A somatogravic illusion may be caused by linear acceleration sensed by the otolith organs, which is perceived as upward or nose-up movement of the aircraft. Credit: SKYbrary

The Head-up or Nose-up Illusion A linear acceleration movement known as the head-up or nose-up illusion occurs during sudden forward acceleration where the pilot's head is forced backward and upward. This linear acceleration is sensed by the otolith organs and is perceived as upward or nose up movement of the aircraft. This sometimes results in the pilot reacting by improperly pushing the nose down. This illusion often happens on takeoff (◻ Fig. 6.14).

The Head-down or Nose-down Illusion An opposite illusion to the Head-up/Nose-up illusion above. Instead of a sudden acceleration, the pilot experiences a sudden deceleration such as applying speed brakes, spoilers or flaps that rapidly slow the forward movement of the aircraft. The resulting linear deceleration is interpreted by the otolith organs as a downward movement, which may result in the pilot abruptly pulling the nose up on the aircraft and possibly causing it to stall. This illusion may happen on landing when applying the flaps and lowering the gear and airspeed simultaneously.

6.2.9.4 Spatial Disorientation in the Vestibular System

There are three integrated systems, the vestibular, the somatosensory and the visual system, which work together to determine orientation and movement in space. This information is sent by these different sensory systems along separate neural pathways to the brain, where it is decoded. The vestibular system detects angular acceleration or deceleration position as well as linear movements. The somatosensory system (nerves in the skin, joints, hearing and feelings often referred to as "seat-of-the-pants" senses) are proprioceptors that detect changes in gravity and acceleration/deceleration. The visual system senses position relative to a known point such as the horizon or stars.

Under normal flight conditions, when there is a visual reference to the horizon and ground, the sensory system in the inner ear helps to identify the pitch, roll and yaw movements of the aircraft. When visual contact with the horizon is lost, the vestibular system becomes unreliable. These three streams of information work together to provide a clear indication of the position of the body within the environment. However, when there is conflicting information between the systems such as the loss of visual references, disorientation can present itself. The loss of visual reference to the horizon or ground is a precursor to spatial disorientation. Spatial orientation refers to one's perception of body position in relation to a reference frame such as the ground horizon or another outside object such as an airplane or even the Sun and stars. This loss of position causes unreliable sensory inputs from the vestibular system, indicating positions such as being in a bank, spinning, diving or even feeling inverted.

Spatial disorientation will manifest itself in three ways. First is *unrecognized spatial disorientation*. In this instance, the pilot is unaware that their perception of orientation is incorrect and may unwillingly control the aircraft into a crash, called controlled flight into terrain (CFIT). In this case, the pilot simply maintains control of the aircraft until it strikes the ground. The second condition is *recognized spatial disorientation*. This condition entails a conscious recognition of disorientation and knowledge by the pilot that there is some conflict between the vertical orientation indicated by the flight instruments and the vestibular senses of balance and motion. Previously in this section, we discussed the vestibular illusions apparent in recognized spatial disorientation, yet we were able to maintain outside references to the horizon or ground. In cases of recognized spatial disorientation, the reference to the horizon or ground is gone.

The third condition is the most dangerous and is known as *incapacitating spatial disorientation*. With incapacitating spatial disorientation, the pilot experiences such an overwhelming sensation of movement that the pilot cannot orient his or herself by using the visual clues of the aircraft instruments. This condition invokes a sense of helplessness and the inability to properly maintain control of the aircraft. The National Transportation Safety Board (NTSB) concluded that John F Kennedy Jr suffered from this type of spatial disorientation due to his lack of visual reference clues while flying at night and entering the fog bank, leading to his subsequent crash.

6.2.10 Can You Trust the Vestibular Senses in Flight?

A method used to train pilots to recognize that their vestibular senses cannot be relied upon with a loss of the horizon is the use of the Barany Chair (◘ Fig. 6.15). This chair was developed by Hungarian physiologist Robert Bárány and is used in aerospace physiology training for student pilots. This device confirms the conflicts between the visual and vestibular senses when a visual impairment occurs. A pilot can experience this condition without being put in danger by performing training exercises in the chair.

A pilot, or anyone, is placed in the chair in a vertical position, head up and blindfolded. The chair is then spun in a circular motion on the vertical axis. After a period of rotation, the occupant is asked questions such as what direction you are turning or how fast you are turning, all while remaining blindfolded and in the chair. After the chair is stopped and the blindfold is removed, the occupant is asked to point to a person holding a sign in front of the occupant. This device may also be used to test an individual's ability to perform cognitive tasks after spinning in the chair. Pilots training in this chair

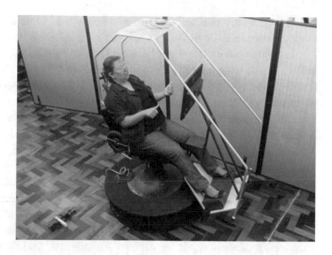

soon experience the unreliable sensory responses caused by the conflicts between the vestibular and ocular organs, which is key to maintaining one's orientation in space. Additionally, the Barany Chair is sometimes used to test the effectiveness of drugs used to counteract the effects of motion sickness.

6.2.11 Nonmedical Treatment for Vertigo

If you experience vertigo or other types of dizziness, it may help to:
- Restrict salt
- take diuretics to reduce the volume of fluid in the body, which could build up in the inner ear
- avoid smoking
- avoid alcohol and caffeine
- if vertigo persists, you should discuss with an Otolaryngologist (Ear, Nose & Throat MD)

6.3 Use of Over-the-Counter and Prescription Drugs

Few pilots realize how much prescription drugs and over-the-counter medications affect their flying skills. Everyone has seen the ads: "Take the little blue pill for..." or "Now the Yellow Tablet can be purchased over the counter." How about the claim "To breathe easy, you can now buy our product, which was formerly only available from a physician"? The fact of the matter is that many drugs that used to be available only by a physician's prescription are now available over the counter. "So what?" you say. It's an over-the-counter (OTC) drug, so it has to be safe, right?

The answer is basically yes, but maybe no. And more importantly, what pilots put into their mouths to mask or prevent medical symptoms of even mild illnesses has a direct impact on the safety of any flight. Officially, the FAA leaves it up to pilots to determine whether they are medically capable to safely fly. As as a pilot, you're as liable for the medical decisions for flight suitability as is the aviation medical examiner (AME).

Let's suppose it's the night before a long-planned flight, and your classic airplane is polished and ready to go. Slowly, you realize that your sinuses are running and you have a mild cough. What should you do? Cancel the trip, find a copilot, or do what many unthinking pilots do? In the end, you follow the last option and go to the local pharmacy to get some non-prescription OTC remedies (see Aside for FAA/CFR guidelines on this issue). A little Nyquil will assure a good night's sleep, and some decongestants can help with the sniffles. With the easing of symptoms, it's tempting to ignore your physical condition and fly. Here's the problem: Nyquil contains 10% alcohol, so it must be taken eight or more hours before a flight, and other ingredients, combined with deconges-tants, can cause dizziness, excessive stimulation, sedation and other undesirable side effects. You need to realize that while you might feel okay at sea level with the OTC meds in your system, that doesn't mean that you'll feel the same at 2,500 feet, or 5,000 feet. Eustachian tubes in the inner ear may be inflamed and literally trap air and fluid in the middle ear, a situation that may produce severe pain and is capable of causing the "leans", or vertigo.

6

Aside

Title 14 CFR § 61.53, Prohibition on Operations During Medical Deficiency

Operations that require a medical certifi-cate. Except as provided in paragraph (b) of this section, a person who holds a current medical certificate issued under part 67 of this chapter shall not act as pilot in com-mand, or in any other capacity as a required pilot flight crewmember, while that person:

1. Knows or has reason to know of any medical condition that would make the person unable to meet the require-ments for the medical certificate neces-sary for the pilot operation; or
2. Is taking medication or receiving other treatment for a medical condition that

results in the person being unable to meet the requirements for the medical certifi-cate necessary for the pilot operation.

Title 14 CFR § 91.17 Alcohol or Drugs
Additionally, FAR 91.17 prohibits the use of "any drug that affects the person's faculties in any way contrary to safety" (AMAS Medication Database). FAR 61.53, 67.113, 67.213, 67.313 and 91.17 preclude flying while having a con-dition or taking a medication that might affect flight safety. However, there is no offi-cial FAA "list" of drugs that is available to the public. Because FAR 91.17 doesn't include the names of the prohibited drugs, there is no requirement that the drugs being taken be made known to the FAA. Therefore, OTC drugs are often mistakenly considered safe for use while flying.

6.3.1 Commonly Used Drugs

The point is that virtually *all* drugs have the potential to cause adverse side effects. That's one reason why so many medications carry the generic warning to avoid operating heavy machinery or motor vehicles while using the drug. These warnings have obviously

Drug category	1990-1997	1998-2002	2003-2007	2008-2012	Total for study period 1990-2014
Sedating antihistamines	5.6%	8.2%	8.3%	9.9%	7.5%
Nonsedating over-the-counter drugs	4.6%	6.8%	6.2%	7.3%	5.9%
Cardiovascular drugs	2.4%	4.2%	8.0%	12.4%	5.7%
Antidepressants	1.0%	4.5%	5.8%	5.3%	3.5%
Illicit drugs	2.3%	2.9%	2.9%	3.8%	2.8%
Sedating pain relievers	1.0%	2.4%	2.6%	4.4%	2.2%
Diet aids	1.2%	2.4%	2.0%	1.2%	1.6%
Benzodiazepines	1.3%	1.1%	0.8%	2.0%	1.3%
Other drugs	0.2%	1.5%	2.1%	1.9%	1.2%
Nonsedating pain relievers	0.6%	0.1%	2.6%	1.7%	1.1%
Blood thinners	1.6%	0.5%	0.1%	1.3%	1.0%
Anti-seizure drugs	0.7%	0.1%	0.6%	1.0%	0.6%
Prostate/erectile dysfunction drugs	0.0%	0.2%	0.8%	1.6%	0.5%
Anti-infective drugs	0.2%	0.7%	0.5%	0.6%	0.4%
Cholesterol lowering drugs	0.1%	0.0%	0.0%	2.0%	0.4%
Other psychotropic drugs	0.2%	0.3%	0.7%	0.8%	0.4%
Migraine drugs	0.3%	0.4%	0.4%	0.3%	0.4%
Prescription sleep aids	0.0%	0.0%	0.2%	1.5%	0.3%
Nausea and vertigo drugs	0.2%	0.1%	0.3%	0.3%	0.2%
Other neurologic drugs	0.1%	0.0%	0.4%	0.6%	0.2%
Oral diabetes drugs	0.0%	0.0%	0.1%	1.0%	0.2%
Emphysema and asthma drugs	0.2%	0.2%	0.0%	0.2%	0.1%

◘ Fig. 6.16 This graphic shows the proportion of pilots with positive findings in certain drug categories and recent trends in positive findings. Each row in the table represents the percentage of pilots in a NTSB study with one or more positive toxicology findings in that category for each time period. Credit: NTSB

greater significance for flying. While some individuals experience no side effects with a drug, others may be noticeably affected. Since each person's response is different, the FAA must consider the worst possible reaction to a drug in evaluating the decision to allow flight duties (◘ Fig. 6.16).

Some of the most commonly used OTC drugs, antihistamines and decongestants have the potential to cause some of the most noticeable side effects and may well be disqualifying as a result. The symptoms associated with common upper respiratory infections, even a bad cold, will usually suppress a pilot's desire to fly, and treating symptoms with a drug that causes side effects only compounds the problem. Some of the more common side effects are drowsiness, dizziness, changes in vision and increased nervousness. Antihistamines (◘ Fig. 6.17) can react with other medications, especially those used to treat diabetes, heart disease and high blood pressure [10].

Manufacturers of these antihistamines will often add a decongestant to the compound, which may contain pseudoephedrine. Decongestants can raise blood pressure

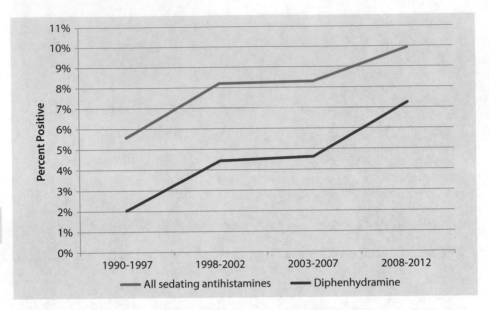

□ **Fig. 6.17**   Recent trends in positive toxicology findings for sedating antihistamines in pilots.
Credit: NTSB

or stimulate fast heart rhythms. Pilots with any of the above diseases should consult their doctor prior to taking such medicines. Fortunately, the previously prescription-only drug Claritin is approved by the FAA for flight and is now available as an OTC drug. The only caveat here is that Claritin, like every drug, prescription or OTC, must be tolerated well. If it isn't, the pilot must report that fact to his or her AME and not use the drug prior to flight.

Allegra (fexofenadine), Claritin (loratadine) and Hismanal (astemizole) are noted to be non-sedating and *are* allowed by the FAA, even though you still might not be legal to fly under FAR 61.53. Remember, a bad head cold may be a "medical deficiency" under the regulations (AOPA Pilot Resources Medical Resources Medications Database). You should be aware that the forms of Allegra and Claritin such as Allegra-D, Zyrtec-D and Claritin-D contain a decongestant and could cause problems for patients with allergies and heart disease. Remember, any drug that produces drowsiness or other central nervous system effects, as well as experimental or investigational drugs are prohibited. These medications include narcotic analgesics, stimulants, sedatives, hypnotics, amphetamines, barbiturates, anti-anxiety drugs, muscle relaxants, tranquilizers and cough syrups with codeine. One of the most widely prescribed cough syrups with antihistamine and often codeine is Promethazine. Promethazine relieves itchy eyes/nose/throat, runny nose and sneezing. Codeine is added as an opioid cough suppressant that affects a certain part of the brain, reducing the urge to cough.

If your illness is serious enough to require medicine, it is serious enough to prevent you from flying. OTC drugs do not usually "cure" your symptoms but hide them for a while until your immune system does its job. When taking these drugs, you will most assuredly not be at your best level of performance. All OTC drugs have side effects and take many forms, including dizziness, disturbance of vision, impairment of judgment and drowsiness. To counteract these effects, pilots often take stimulant caffeine products, which when mixed usually make a person hyperactive.

The bottom line is that pilots should read and pay special attention to label warnings on any drug. They should not fly while using any medication, prescription or OTC that carries a label precaution or warning that it "may cause drowsiness" or advises the user "be careful when driving a motor vehicle or operating machinery". This applies even if the label states "until you know how the medication affects you", or if the pilot has used the medication before with no apparent adverse effect. Such medications can cause impairment even when the pilot feels alert and unimpaired.

Among physician-administered drugs, streptomycin is widely used to treat bacterial infections. One of the most concerning side effects to pilots is *ototoxicity*. Ototoxicity is the condition of being toxic to the ear, specifically the cochlea or auditory nerve and sometimes the vestibular system, possibly causing transient or permanent deafness. The vestibular portion of the cranial nerve (the vestibulocochlear nerve) can be affected, resulting in a common side effect of vertigo (Kubo et al. [11]).

6.3.2 Controlled Substances

Previously, we discussed the vestibulo-ocular reflex (VOR) where the eyes move opposite the head direction when rapid head movement occurs. The VOR is a central part of the sensori-motor system. It carries the information from the labyrinth (inner ear organs responsible for balance and hearing) over the vestibular nerve and its area in the brainstem to the eye muscles. The VOR transmits information from the semicircular canals via the vestibular nerve, the brainstem nuclei and the vestibular projection to the nuclei of the three eye muscles (three-neuron arc, oculomotor crus) (Masao [12]). A person's sense of balance is related to labyrinth function, the visual system and cervical deep sensibility. These senses work in an interconnected manner to control visual motor activity and provide spatial orientation in all positions and during head movement.

Why are we revisiting a discussion of the VOR? Like so many systems in the body, the VOR can also be affected by OTCs, especially antihistamines, blood pressure medications, pain relievers and sleep aids.

» Further analysis of toxicology findings and pilot characteristics indicated that drug usage was not evenly distributed among all study pilots. For example, a comparison of findings by pilot age indicated that use of all drugs, potentially impairing drugs, drugs used to treat potentially impairing medical conditions, and controlled substances was more common among older study pilots. The increasing trends with age were statistically significant for each of these drug categories. ([13], p. 23)

Recently, a study (Weiler et al. [14]) was conducted on the effects of pilots' use of all drugs for over 22 years, and included 6,677 pilots involved in fatal accidents and potentially impairing drugs, drugs used to treat potentially impairing conditions, drugs designated as controlled substances and illicit drugs (◘ Figs. 6.18 and 6.19). The most common potentially impairing drug pilots used was diphenhydramine, an antihistamine that is an active ingredient in many OTC allergy formulations, cold medicines

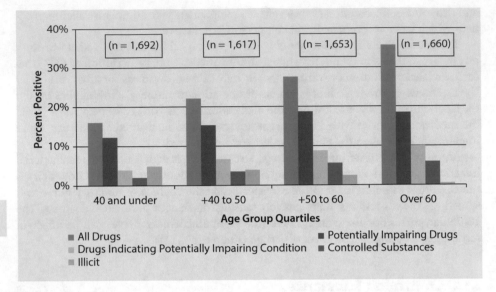

□ **Fig. 6.18** Potentially impairing drugs and conditions, controlled substances and illicit drugs by pilot age group. According to the NTSB Safety Study, sedating antihistamines are the most commonly detected medication in fatal accidents. The study found that pilots in 40% of the 200 fatal accidents studied tested positive for some form of drug. Credit: NTSB

and sleep aids in the US. Brands such as Benadryl, Allergy Benadryl, Diphenhist, Wal-Dryl, Nytol, Unisom and ZzzQuil are among those impairing OTC drugs. Although widely available in the US in multiple over-the-counter formulations intended to treat allergies and colds and be used as a sleep aid, diphenhydramine causes significant sedation and is one of the few individual drugs that has been tested and found to significantly degrade operator performance. Weiler's study found that a *single dose of diphenhydramine* impaired driving ability more than a blood alcohol concentration of 0.100 gm/dL in a driving simulator. Based on this study of fatally injured pilots, the use of diphenhydramine in the population may be continuing to increase, suggesting a potential safety issue in transportation. Often, drugs with diphenhydramine as an active ingredient state, "Be careful when driving a motor vehicle or operating machinery." This may not be sufficient information to clearly warn users of the risks associated with this drug.

6.3.3 **Summary**

Healthy audible (ears), visual (eyes) and cognitive (brain) functions are your best prevention against symptoms of vertigo and spells of dizziness. Keeping your body in good physical shape combined with exercise is critical to maintaining the heath of your sensory systems. Use of training devices can help to identify conflicts in your sensory systems. Even so, don't forget that the best method to avoid vertigo and spatial disorientation is to recognize the onset of the symptoms and trust your flight instruments.

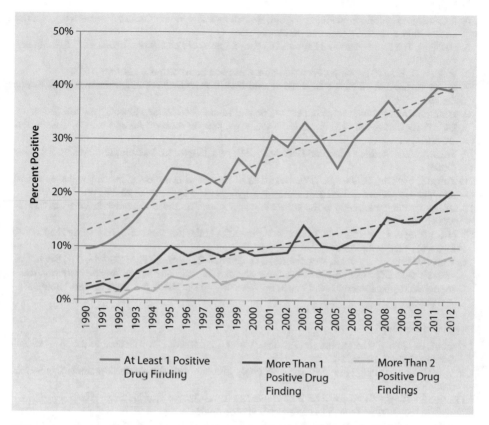

Fig. 6.19 Percentages of study pilots with at least one positive and multiple toxicology findings.
Credit: NTSB

Review Questions
1. Can the use of drugs, alcohol, or caffeine affect the vestibular system? How?
2. Give an example of a somatogravic illusion
3. Give an example of a vestibular illusion
4. What functions do the semicircular canals sense?
5. What functions do the Otolith organs sense?
6. Name the senses which contribute to the Vestibulo-Ocular reflex
7. What purpose do the Cilia nerve cells serve?

References

1. Dominguez, C., Vidulich, M., Vogel, E., McMillan, G.: Situation awareness: papers and annotated bibliography. Armstrong Laboratory, Human System Center, ref. AL/CF-TR-1994-0085 (1994)
2. Maurino, D., Reason, J., Johnston, N., Lee, R.: Beyond Aviation Human Factors. Ashgate Publishing Limited, Aldershot (2000)
3. Salas, E., Maurino, D.: Human Factors in Aviation. Academic Press, Burlington (2010)

4. Rasmussen, J.: Information Processing and Human-machine Interaction: an Approach to Cognitive Engineering. Elsevier Science Ltd, New York (1986)
5. Hellier, J.: The Five Senses and Beyond, the Encyclopedia of Perception. ABC-CLIO, LLC, Santa Barbara (2016)
6. O'Brien, D.: How to Develop a Perfect Memory. Pavilion Books Limited, London (1993)
7. Burch, N.: Learning a New Skill is Easier Said than Done. Gordon Training International, Solana Beach
8. Desmond, A.: Vestibular Function: Evaluation and Treatment. Thieme Medical, New York (2004)
9. FAA: Pilot's Handbook of Aeronautical Knowledge. Federal Aviation Administration, Washington, DC (2016)
10. Stedman, T.L.: Stedman's Medical Dictionary, 28th edn. Lippincott, Williams, and Wilkins, Baltimore (2006)
11. Kubo, T., Igarashi, M., Jensen, D.W., Wright, W.K.: Head and eye movements following vestibular stimulus in squirrel monkeys. ORL J Otorhinolaryngol Relat Spec. **43**(1), 26–38 (1981)
12. Ito, M.: Cerebellar learning in the vestibule-ocular reflex. Trends in Cognitive Sciences. **2**(9), 313–321 (1998)
13. NTSB, Drug use trends in aviation: assessing the risk of pilot impairment. Safety Study 2014, NTSB/SS-14/01, PB2014-108827.
14. Weiler, J.M., Bloomfield, J.R., Woodworth, G.G., Grant, A.R., Layton, T.A., McKenzie, D.R., Baker, T.W., Watson, G.S.: Effects of fexofenadine, diphenhydramine, and alcohol on driving performance. A randomized, placebo-controlled trial in the Iowa driving simulator. Ann. Intern. Med. **132**(5), 354–363 (2000)

Suggested Reading

Campbell, R.D., Bagshaw, M.: Human Performance and Limitations in Aviation, 2nd edn. Blackwell Science Limited, Oxford (1999)
Green, R.G., Muir, H., et al.: Human Factors for Pilots, 2nd edn. Ashgate Publishing Limited, Aldershot (1996)
NTSB Accident Report NYC99MA178: JFK Jr. Piper Saratoga – Spatial disorientation (1999)
SKYbrary, A310, Quebec, Canada: Somatogravic illusion (2008)
SKYbrary, A320 Bahrain Airport Kingdom of Bahrain: Somatogravic illusion (2000)

Communication

© Springer Nature Switzerland AG 2020
E. Seedhouse et al., *Human Factors in Air Transport*,
https://doi.org/10.1007/978-3-030-13848-6_7

Learning Objectives

After completing this chapter, you should be able to

- Describe some of the factors that compromise effective communication
- Describe two accidents caused by ineffective communication
- Briefly explain the rationale of the ICAO Language Proficiency Requirements
- List three characteristics of the LPR and explain how they enhance communication
- Explain what is meant by the phrase "Power Distance"
- Briefly describe three environmental variables that may affect pilot-ATC communication
- Explain how assertiveness or its lack thereof can compromise effective communication
- Understand what factor was implicated in the Air Florida Flight 90 accident
- Explain what is meant by "fluency" and "structure" in the context of communication
- In reference to Zastrow's model, list four factors that may cause communication to break down

7   7.1   Introduction

Given the importance of communication in the aviation industry, it is not surprising that this particular human factor is among the most frequently studied in human factors programs. In every aspect of aviation, training to improve and refine communication skills is accepted as a critical part of ensuring flight safety. But what exactly is communication?

At the most basic level, communication can be either formal or informal. Formal communication implies that a record is made of what is said, whereas informal communication requires no record. Another criterion for defining communication is whether it is spoken or written. This is important because spoken communication is more likely to be misinterpreted than written communication. In the aviation industry, communication is formalized, defined and regulated. On the subject of written communication, written correspondence parameters are defined in the Federal Aviation Regulations (FARs), a repository that includes important information such as notices to airmen (NOTAMs) and airworthiness directives (ADs) [1]. Spoken communication between aircrew is governed by a highly restricted and structured subset of English language, whose aim is to reduce error and enhance safety. This structure—which includes written protocols, graphical protocols and verbal protocols—helps reduce ambiguities, limit variances and establish clear regulations governing the meaning of words and phrases.

Despite the rigor that guides communication in the aviation industry, a significant number of accidents are still caused by a failure to apply verbal protocols. These accidents can be caused by crew using the wrong information, losing situational awareness or failing to build a shared model of the situation they find themselves in. Accidents may also be caused by a myriad other reasons, such as those presented in ◘ Table 7.1.

7.2   Accident Analysis

To illustrate the consequences of failed communication, it is instructive to examine some of the more prominent accidents that have been caused by this particular human factor. We'll begin with Avianca Flight 52 (◘ Fig. 7.1).

Table 7.1 Factors affecting communication

Ambiguous phraseology	Partial readback
Block transmission	Pilot accent
Controller distraction	Pilot distraction
Controller fatigue	Pilot fatigue
Controller high speech rate	Pilot high speech rate
Controller non-standard phraseology	Pilot non-standard phraseology
Controller workload	Pilot workload
Frequency change	Untimely transmission
Message content inaccurate	Similar call-sign
Language problems	Long message

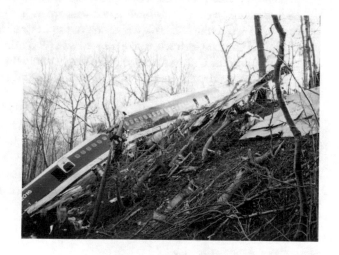

Fig. 7.1 Picture of the wreckage of Avianca Flight 52 in Cove Neck, New York. Credit: NTSB/FAA

— **On January 25, 1990, Avianca Flight 92** was in a holding pattern near its New York destination. Due to bad weather, the aircraft had been circling for more than 90 minutes and was running low on fuel and the situation was urgent. Unfortunately for the passengers and crew, when the flight was passed from regional to local ATC, the local ATC was not informed that the aircraft had insufficient fuel to reach the alternative airport. Making matters worse, the crew did not specifically state there was a fuel emergency. The outcome of all this flawed communication was that the aircraft was given a landing pattern for which it had insufficient fuel and its engines flamed out. 65 of the 149 passengers and 8 of the 9 crew were killed.

- **On January 13, 1982, Air Florida Flight 90** was preparing to take off from Washington National Airport, but conditions were wintry and the aircraft's de-icing system was not working effectively. Making matters worse, the engine anti-icing system had not been activated, which meant the instruments did not provide correct readings. Oblivious to this, the crew oblivious applied the power they thought they needed to take off. After they had traveled more than half a mile longer than usual, the first officer knew they were in trouble and voiced his concern to the captain. The captain ignored his first officer and the aircraft crashed into the 14th Street Bridge, killing 78.
- **On October 8, 2001, a Cessna Citation CJ2** jet was given clearance to taxi to its takeoff point at Linate Airport, Milan, Italy. Unfortunately, due to poor communication and lack of correct markings, the Cessna misunderstood the message and proceeded in the wrong direction, crossing the main runway. In its way was SAS Flight 686, a McDonnell Douglas MD-87. The planes collided, killing 118.
- **On September 25, 1978, a Boeing 727 Pacific Southwest Airlines Flight 182** was on its way to San Diego. Nearby was a Cessna piloted by a student and an instructor. Inexplicably, the Cessna made an unauthorized course alteration which put it on collision course with the Boeing 727. In a transmission between ATC and Flight 182, the word "passed" may have been misheard as "passing". This was confirmation to ATC that the 182 crew was aware of the Cessna's location. In reality, the Boeing 727 had no idea where the Cessna was. Two minutes after that fateful transmission, the Cessna struck the 182's right wing. Both aircraft plummeted into a San Diego residential area, killing 135 on the aircraft and 7 on the ground. It was California's deadliest air disaster.
- **On November 12, 1996, Kazakhstan Airlines Flight 1907** was struggling with turbulence, prompting the crew to descend 1,000 feet below its assigned altitude of 15,000 feet. This maneuver placed Flight 1907 on a collision course with Saudi Arabian Airlines Flight 763. Since no one onboard Flight 1907 except the radio operator understood English, the crew was mostly reliant on ATC communication. The ultimate outcome of the language barrier was the collision of the two aircraft and the loss of 349 passengers and crew.

7.3 Standardization

In addition to this list, we can add the Tenerife accident (◘ Fig. 7.2) that was covered in ▶ Chap. 1. In light of these incidents, what can be done to improve communication? The aviation industry recognized just how important communication was some time ago, and in 1951 the International Civil Aviation Organization (ICAO) decided to use English as the international aviation language. In establishing English as the aviation language, ICAO ensured a high level of consistency and accuracy in air-to-ground and ground-to air-communication. It helped reduce communication error, language problems and comprehension difficulties. Another level of standardization in the application of Aviation English is its structure.

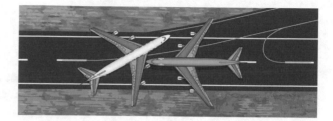

◻ Fig. 7.2 Animation of the collision, with the taxiing Pan Am plane (left) attempting to turn away from the KLM plane (right) on its takeoff run. Credit: SafetyCard

7.3.1 Aviation English

Aviation English is rather different than regular English since it features a highly specialized vocabulary and a language that emphasizes very specific pronunciation. This language can be categorized as standard *aviation phraseology* and *plain language*. The former is the aviation-specific language used by ATC and pilots, while the latter "plain language" is exactly that—the language we use in everyday communication. But it is one thing to learn the vocabulary and another to actually be able to communicate. To that end, ICAO established Language Proficiency Requirements (LPR) to minimize miscommunication. The LPR (Appendix VI) includes pronunciation, structure, vocabulary, fluency, comprehension and interaction, and the proficiency in each of these categories is rated from Level 1 to Level 6. Under these requirements, pilots flying international and air traffic controllers serving international airports must achieve a Level 4 or higher. And, since language is a perishable skill, these language requirements are reassessed every 36 months. The criteria (adapted from ICAO) are listed below:

- **Pronunciation.** Dialect and/or accent intelligible to the aeronautical community
- **Structure.** Relevant grammatical structures and sentence patterns determined by language functions appropriate to the task
- **Vocabulary.** Vocabulary range and accuracy used sufficiently to communicate effectively
- **Fluency.** Produces stretches of language at an appropriate tempo
- **Comprehension.** Comprehension accurate in common, concrete and work-related topics, and the accent used is sufficiently intelligible for the international community
- **Interactions.** Responses are immediate, appropriate and informative

For non-English speakers, achieving the Level 4 requirement is a challenge due to speech structures, grammar and vocabulary. Also, the intonation of certain words and phrases and rapid speech rate also cause problems for those learning to be proficient in ICAO English. Further, despite the commonality of the language and the high language proficiency required, barriers to effective communication still exist. Remember, the ICAO language requirements were implemented in 1951 and since then there have been dozens of accidents that were caused or partly caused by miscommunication. Most of these barriers occur in communication between pilots and ATC and between ATC and pilots. Before we discuss some of these barriers, it is important to understand what effective communication is. One way to do this is to use a simple model as follows:

» Sender (Encodes) > Message > Receiver (Decodes) > Receiver Becomes Sender and Encodes > Message > Receiver (Decodes)

(Zastrow, 2001) [2]

In Zastrow's model, effective communication may break down if the message is not encoded or decoded correctly. This may occur for a number of reasons:
- Noise, static
- Multiple communications
- Fatigue, stress
- Distractions
- Incomplete message
- Ambiguous wording
- Lack of credibility
- Lack of rapport
- Thinking in personal terms
- Jargon
- Boring

7.4 Assertiveness in Communication

Now that we are armed with the basics of the communication process, we can examine this in a practical context and take a look at what happens in the cockpit and the control tower. Over the years, research has revealed that communication has remained a consistent and persistent problem in the aviation world, with language variables highly correlated with individual pilot performance and error rates [3–5]. This happens for a number of reasons. For example, communication may be compromised by the interaction (or lack thereof) between the captain and copilot. Such a scenario may occur when a captain is an especially assertive individual and the copilot is a passive individual. In such a situation, the copilot may feel uncomfortable speaking up in the face of a contingency. Let's not forget that the FAR 91.3 states the following: "The pilot in command of an aircraft is directly responsible for, and is the final authority as to, the operation of that aircraft". In other words, the copilot is essentially a subordinate member of the flight crew who must tread a fine line between speaking up when required and not being overly assertive when doing so. An example? Consider the case of the Air Florida Flight 90 incident that occurred in January 1992 [6]:
- CAM-1 Captain's Cockpit Area Microphone
- CAM-2 First Officer's Cockpit Area Microphone RDO-1 Captain's Radio TWR
- Washington National Tower

- 15:59:16 CAM-1 Given.
- 15:59:16 CAM-2 Bleeds?
- 15:59:17 CAM-1 They're off.
- 15:59:18 CAM-2 Strobes, external lights.
- 15:59:18 CAM-1 On.

- 15:59:19 CAM-2 Anti-skid?
- 15:59:19 CAM-1 On.
- 15:59:21 CAM-2 Transponder?
- 15:59:21 CAM-1 On.
- 15:59:24 TWR Palm 90 cleared for takeoff.
- 15:59:28 TWR No delay on departure if you will, traffic's two and a half out for the runway.
- 15:59:32 CAM-1 Okay, your throttles.
- 15:59:35 [SOUND OF ENGINE SPOOLUP]
- 15:59:49 CAM-1 Holler if you need the wipers.
- 15:59:51 CAM-1 It's spooled. Real cold, real cold.
- 15:59:58 CAM-2 God, look at that thing. That don't seem right, does it? Uh, that's not right.
- 16:00:09 CAM-1 Yes it is, there's eighty.
- 16:00:10 CAM-2 Naw, I don't think that's right. Ah, maybe it is.
- 16:00:21 CAM-1 Hundred and twenty.
- 16:00:23 CAM-2 I don't know
- 16:00:31 CAM-1 Vee-one. Easy, vee-two.
- 16:00:39 [SOUND OF STICKSHAKER STARTS AND CONTINUES UNTIL IMPACT]
- 16:00:41 TWR Palm 90 contact departure control.
- 16:00:45 CAM-1 Forward, forward, easy. We only want five hundred.
- 16:00:48 CAM-1 Come on forward....forward, just barely climb.
- 16:00:59 CAM-1 Stalling, we're falling!
- 16:01:00 CAM-2 Larry, we're going down, Larry....
- 16:01:01 CAM-1 I know it.
- 16:01:01 [SOUND OF IMPACT]

In this accident, the copilot noticed that something was amiss with the engine instruments, but the captain ignored the copilot's concerns and proceeded with the takeoff. The copilot was persistent and stated the issue as "not being right" no less than six times. The captain, however, was seemingly oblivious to the copilot's concerns and did not use or act upon the conflicting information presented to him by the first officer. What should the first officer have done differently in this situation? He could have been more assertive to the extent of calling an abort. So why didn't the first officer do this? Perhaps he was afraid of job repercussions by being assertive to a more experienced captain? The truth is, we don't know, but what we do know is that the accident, which killed 70 of the 74 passengers and crew, was caused by deficient communication.

7.4.1 Power Distance

Since the Air Florida 90 accident, the development of crew resource management (CRM) has helped reduced the chance of similar circumstances being repeated, but the power distance (PD) barrier still exists more than a quarter of a century later [7, 8]. In

◘ Fig. 7.3 Military ATC. Credit: USAF

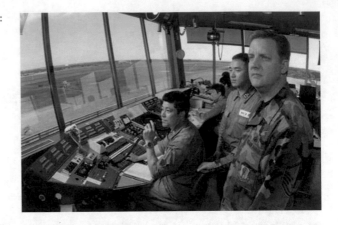

its practical application, PD describes the unequal power relationship in the cockpit. In some cultures, PD is high, which means insubordinates feel uncomfortable speaking up and are therefore unwilling to make inputs concerning the decisions of their superiors. Research has shown that countries such as Denmark, Norway and the United States scored very low on the PD scale, which means that in these countries, subordinates are more likely to speak up in the event of an issue. Conversely, countries such as Taiwan and the Philippines have very high PD scores, which means subordinates in these countries are much less likely to question a superior.

7.4.2 Pilot-ATC Communication

Now that we have covered some of the problems of pilot-to-pilot communication, it is instructive to consider some of the deficiencies of the communication process between ATC (◘ Fig. 7.3) and the cockpit [8]. In many of the accident scenarios in which pilot-ATC miscommunication was deemed a factor, a common thread has been the language barrier. You might think this shouldn't be a problem since English is the international language of aviation, but language proficiency varies greatly among pilots and controllers. This is because the command of the English language can be affected by such variables as dialects, accents and/or simple misinterpretation. Making matters worse is the particular phraseology used by US crews, which can sometimes sound incomprehensible to foreign crews. Other compounding factors include environmental variables such as *clipping, masking* and *blocking*. The first of these, clipping, may occur when a microphone is unkeyed before a transmission is complete. This can lead to broken and incomplete (and frustrating!) communication. Masking is when a transmission is distorted by noise. This environmental variable is more common during the takeoff and climb phases and can cause misunderstandings, requiring that instructions be repeated. Blocking is simply having someone "step on" the frequency. When this happens, the transmission is blocked. One final barrier to pilot-ATC communication is the use of words that sound similar. For example, "five thousand" may sound similar to "nine thousand", especially when there is a lot of background noise.

7.5 **Summary**

The importance of communication in aviation is critical, because this particular human factor has such an impact on safety. It is therefore imperative that efforts are made to enhance the quality of communication. This can be achieved via the proactive creation of safety nets, improved quality assurance, enhancing language proficiency and increasing awareness of all the myriad factors that can compromise communication.

Key Terms
AD - Airworthiness Directive

ATC - Air Traffic Control

CRM - Crew Resource Management

FAR - Federal Aviation Regulations

ICAO - International Civil Aviation Organization

LPR - Language Proficiency Requirements

NOTAM - Notices to Airmen

PDP - Power Distance

Review Questions
1. Briefly describe three factors that compromise effective communication
2. List three accidents caused by ineffective communication and in each case identify the specific failure in communication that caused the accident
3. What are the key features of the ICAO Language Proficiency Requirements?
4. Explain what is meant by the phrase "Power Distance"
5. Describe two environmental variables that may affect pilot-ATC communication
6. Explain how assertiveness can adversely affect effective communication
7. Explain what factor was implicated in the Air Florida Flight 90 accident
8. Explain what is meant by "fluency" in the context of communication
9. In reference to Zastrow's model, list four factors that may cause communication to break down
10. What is meant by "blocking"?

References

1. Code of Federal Regulations: Federal aviation regulations [electronic version]. Available at http://ecfr.gpoaccess.gov (2004)
2. Zastrow, C.: Social Work with Groups: Using the Class as a Group Leadership Laboratory, 5th edn. Brooks/Cole, Pacific Grove (2001)
3. Aviation Today: Special Reports: Report on aviation safety. language barriers. Retrieved 31 May 2004 from http://www.aviationtoday.com/reports/V.htm (2004)

4. Connell, L.: Pilot and controller communications issues. In: Kanki, B.G., Prinzo, O.V. (eds.) Proceedings of the Methods and Metrics of Voice Communication Workshops. U.S. Federal Aviation Administration, Office of Aviation Medicine, Washington, DC (1995)
5. Helmreich, R.L., Wilhelm, J.A., Klinect, J.R., Merritt, A.C.: Culture, Error, and Crew Resource Management. The University of Texas at Austin. Department of Psychology, Austin (2001)
6. PlaneCrashInfo.com: Cockpit voice recording transcript of Air Florida Flight 90. Retrieved 14 May 2004 from http://www.planecrashinfo.com/cvr820113.htm (2004)
7. Kirby, J.: Crew resource management (CRM) PowerPoint presentation. A presentation of the Salt Lake City Flight Standards District Office (FSDO) (1997)
8. Cooper, G.E., White, M.D., Lauber, J.K. (eds.): Resource Management on the Flightdeck: Proceedings of a NASA/Industry Workshop (NASA CP-2120). NASA-Ames Research Center, Moffett Field (1980)

Suggested Reading

DynamicFlight.com: Effective communication. Retrieved 31 May 2004 from http://www.dynamicflight.com/avcfibook/communication (2004)
Orlady, H.W., Orlady, L.M.: Human Factors in Multi-crew Flight Operations. Ashgate, Brookfield (1999)
Secretary of Aviation Report on Tenerife Crash: KLM, B-747, PH-BUF and Pan Am B-747 N736 collision at Tenerife Airport Spain on 27 March 1977. Retrieved from http://www.aviationcrm.com/TENERIFE.htm (1978)

7

Training

© Springer Nature Switzerland AG 2020
E. Seedhouse et al., *Human Factors in Air Transport*,
https://doi.org/10.1007/978-3-030-13848-6_8

Learning Objectives

After completing this chapter, you should be able to
- Describe the principles of positive and negative training transfer
- Explain the principles and evolution of Crew Resource Management
- Describe transcockpit authority gradient
- Describe the effects of attitudes and persuasion
- Describe flight training and types of simulation
- List some enhancements to training as a product of advancements in technology

8.1 Training

How is training different than teaching? Both terms are often used interchangeably, but there are differences. Teaching seeks to convey knowledge, while the intent of training is to develop one's skills. Acquiring the knowledge and skills used in aviation requires a great deal of teaching and learning, but training a fledgling aviator to understand how concepts as seemingly uncomplicated as how checklist discipline or sterile cockpit might affect the safety of a flight is a process that begins in a classroom and continues throughout an aviator's career. A long list of human factors-related examples is present in every flight department. But learning does not only happen at flight school. Those in the aviation career fields will find teachers from the earliest days in their careers to the end.

8.1.1 Training Principles

Education and training are both aspects of teaching. Generally, education precedes training. Education is begun at an early age, with youngsters learning the very basics of math, language and scientific principles that will be expanded upon throughout a typical school career. This process of gaining knowledge, skills, values and even attitudes establish the foundation upon which more precise abilities used to perform a job are built (◘ Fig. 8.1).

A common refrain among high school students is *Why do we need to learn algebra? We'll never use it in the real world!* Algebra is a basic building block of sorts. While we may not use actual formulas, algebra is used when planning travel, determining which mobile phone company offers the best deal, or even calculating debt or mortgage payments. Algebra helps people think logically. Similar building blocks make potential employees in need of skillsets more trainable. Attempting to train a worker without an adequate background is like building a house without a foundation. Training builds upon education. The process is aimed at developing specific skills, knowledge and attitudes to be used in jobs that require high levels of skill.

In the aviation community as well as many other high-tech career fields, motor skills and the ability to communicate clearly are very important. Teaching these skills requires its own skillset. A flight school, for example, must differentiate between pilots who have exceptional knowledge versus those who have great skill. The difference? A newly certificated pilot has skills. A star basketball player has skills. But knowledge requires depth

◘ Fig. 8.1 Education and training are both aspects of teaching. Generally, education precedes training. Credit: Alex Pereslavtsev

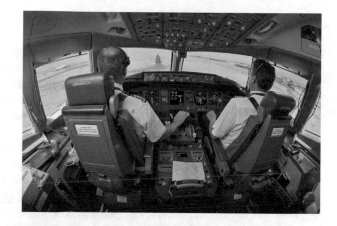

◘ Fig. 8.2 Delta Air Lines Boeing 737-800. Credit: Delta Airlines

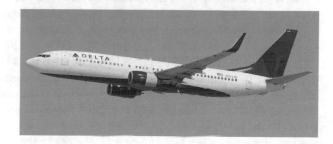

of experience, such as that possessed by a top basketball coach, an instructor or an evaluator pilot.

Another principle of training is that of training transfer. What is learned in one set of circumstances can apply or be used in another situation. For example, some aspects of learning to drive a new car might be made easier if the driver has owned a similar or earlier model of that car. What was difficult to learn in one case transfers to another in a positive manner, allowing the driver to adapt more quickly. When a pilot moves from one Boeing aircraft type to another, or from one Airbus type to another Airbus, cockpit layouts and procedures will already be familiar. The improvement in learning time resulting from earlier training and experience is referred to as positive transfer. Alternatively, negative transfer can complicate learning. The locations of switches and handles between dissimilar automobiles or aircraft can interfere with learning to operate the new machinery.

Is it possible to eliminate negative transfer? Certainly, negative transfer can be a problem, especially with the prevalence of airline mergers and the integration of aircraft fleets and crewmembers. Standardization of equipment, cockpit configuration and procedures can all help to minimize negative transfer. Even the introduction of a helpful new system can introduce negative transfer problems. One of the most successful air carriers in the US saw the benefits of operating all aircraft of the same type—the Boeing 737 (◘ Fig. 8.2). While it continues to operate different series of the B-737, including the 737-700, 737-800 and 737-Max, Southwest Airlines pilots with the B-737-type rating can operate all company aircraft with minimal negative transfer concerns.

8.1.2 Crew Resource Management

Humans are susceptible to making mistakes individually and in groups. The complex processes involved in operating commercial aircraft, if accomplished with any degree of safety and efficiency, would seem to be quite the challenge given the human capacity to err. Still, thousands of flights are completed daily without so much as a hiccup. Though commercial aviation is relatively safe today, historically, accident rates were much higher before the development of Crew Resource Management (CRM).

The history of aviation is scattered with accidents, many of which blamed "pilot error" as a causal factor. The International Air Transport Association (IATA) 20th Technical Conference in Istanbul in late 1975 was the turning point in officially recognizing the importance of Human Factors in aviation, recognizing that accidents resulting from pilot error were not due to carelessness or deliberate acts by crewmembers, but rather a series of conditions that put the aircrew in a situation where the probability of making an error was unusually high. In a move to shift away from the tendency of holding pilots responsible when things go wrong, investigators and airline management pursued the answer to the million-dollar question: Why are these errors made?

As mentioned earlier in this book, less than two years later, two Boeing 747 aircraft collided on the Spanish island of Tenerife in the Canary Islands, causing the greatest loss of life in any single accident to date in the history of commercial aviation. The accident was a result of several human factors-related mistakes, including a glaring error made by one of the pilots and not questioned strongly enough by others on his crew. One of the captains erroneously believed he had takeoff clearance, and other crewmembers on his aircraft were not assertive in questioning his move to begin the takeoff without confirming proper clearance. Blanketed in fog, the other aircraft was still facing them on the runway, having missed its turn. The resulting tragedy cost 583 people their lives.

Most plane crashes result not from a single failure or error, but rather from a chain of failures and errors. Over time, the list of accidents illustrating this fact grew to an unignorable point. After the controlled flight into terrain (CFIT) accident of Eastern Airlines Flight 401 in 1972, the accident at Tenerife and United Airlines Flight 173 running out of fuel and crashing after focusing too long on a suspected landing gear malfunction in 1978, the CRM concept was finally born [1, 2]. Initially, CRM stood for Cockpit Resource Management and was focused almost exclusively on the crewmembers on the flight deck—in those days, two pilots and a flight engineer. At that time, CRM concentrated on shaping the individual behavior of crewmembers. Captains were to incorporate input from their other flight deck crewmembers in their decision making, which was quite the change from the usual pattern of "The Captain is in charge—do not question the Captain".

Since then, CRM (◘ Fig. 8.3) has evolved to include nearly everyone who interfaces with the pilots, including flight attendants, maintenance personnel, dispatch, weather, ATC and others. In the early 1980s, United Airlines and KLM Airlines led the global drive toward CRM, emphasizing personality styles and leadership. In 1984, CRM was redefined by Dr. John Lauber as "the effective utilization of all available resources—hardware, software, and liveware—to achieve safe, efficient flight operation" [3]. The liveware, of course, referred to humans. Group decision making was highlighted, recog-

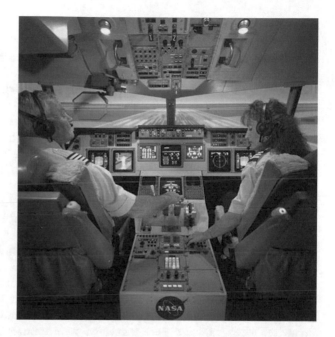

Fig. 8.3 A key platform for learning CRM practices is the flight simulator. This cockpit happens to be the Advanced Cockpit Flight Simulator located at NASA Ames Research Center. Credit: NASA

nizing that others such as cabin crew sometimes have crucial information that, when communicated expeditiously to the flight crew, might prevent an accident.

The most recent evolution of CRM introduced *Threat and Error Management (TEM)* as a prescribed approach for recognizing sources of threats to safety and preventing them from affecting safety of flight as early as possible. A threat might be any condition that complicates the usual tasks, be it internal or external. Internal threats are things within a worker's control, such as being under stress due to a late wakeup or personal issues at home. For example, pilots who show up for a 5 am flight may be fatigued from lack of sleep. External threats are outside of one's control and might include weather, aircraft maintenance issues or last-minute changes in flight plan. Rain or ice will certainly impact takeoff and landing performance. When not properly addressed, threats can cause errors and impact safety. A tired pilot accepting a clearance to land on a shorter runway in the rain without much leeway for the unexpected is an accident waiting to happen.

Assertiveness with respect is a central theme of CRM. Though crewmembers have been trained to speak up and voice concerns about status or a plan of action, the captain is still the final authority and is directly responsible for the safe operation of the aircraft. In CRM training, individuals are taught how to candidly state their concerns immediately without challenging the authority of the pilot in command. A climate of mutual respect is important to ensure success, and hours are spent in simulators and classrooms demonstrating scenarios where the least likely person has key information. Quite often, someone in the chain of events could intervene and prevent an accident. Regardless of the tone set by the captain, all involved with moving an aircraft from one location to another are obligated to voice their concerns on matters of safety.

8.1.3 **Transcockpit Authority Gradient**

The *transcockpit authority gradient* is the balance of perceived authority between subordinates and the designated leader. The captain is the leader of the flight crew, designated by the airline to be "in charge". Personal factors such as the captain's age, gender, experience, appearance, physical size, voice and reputation can impact his or her ability to effectively lead a crew and can even create misperceptions as to which pilot has more informal authority in the cockpit. Preferably, the captain will convey more authority than anyone else on the flight crew, but exuding too much authority can engender problems with CRM. A captain must be mindful not to project too much or too little authority.

The optimal gradient, where the captain is recognized by all as the final authority and the primary decision maker, at the same time that his or her subordinates feel included and part of the decision-making process, is depicted as TAG1 in ◘ Fig. 8.4. A flat gradient, where the second pilot or other crewmembers perceive equal authority in decision making, is depicted as TAG2. While two-way communication is good, a captain should never give up their role as leader. A flat gradient might occur when two pilots of equal experience or rank are paired to fly together. There can only be one final authority. TAG3 depicts a steep authority gradient reflective of pre-CRM behavior, when captains were perceived as domineering, or when subordinates lacked assertiveness. Finally, TAG 4 depicts a reverse or negative gradient—a very dangerous situation. This negative gradient occurs when the captain, designated leader of the flight crew, is not the practical leader. Another crewmember wields too much influence over decision making. This gradient might occur when an experienced first officer corrects a few of the captain's procedures at a new airfield, causing the captain to begin deferring to the first officer on even more matters. It is the captain's responsibility to manage the authority gradient, and should an overly assertive crewmember start pushing decisions unilaterally, the captain should gently remind that crewmember that while their input is welcome, the captain will make the final decision.

8.1.4 **Attitudes and Persuasion**

Many variables affect human performance. People are subject to psychological factors of all types. It should be recognized that different types of flying call for different personality traits. In Tom Wolfe's 1979 book *The Right Stuff*, the world was introduced to the larger-than-life personalities of fighter pilots who would become America's first astronauts. The competitive spirit and fearlessness that defined these men was not unlike the personalities of a typical airline captain pre-CRM. Even today, single-seat fighter aircraft have little need for CRM, though help from the ground can surely be welcome in an emergency when there's time to work a complex problem. Some personality traits are desirable in the civil aviation community, while others may not be optimum when flying with other crewmembers. Today, airline interviews include questions and testing that provide an effective means of assessing pilot personalities and attitudes, allowing companies to weed out those who might not be a good fit or might

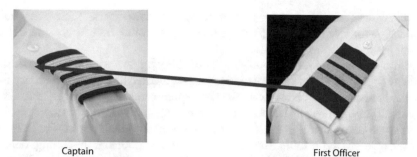

Captain   First Officer
TAG1. Ideal authority gradient. Nominal command authority.

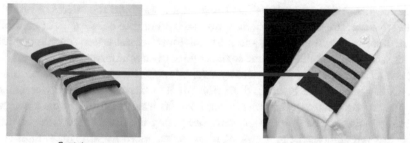

Captain   First Officer
TAG2. Flat authority gradient. Equal decision-making: less than ideal

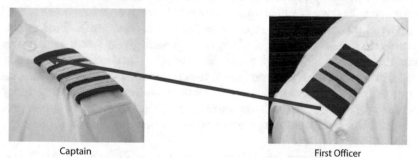

Captain   First Officer
TAG3. Steep authority gradient. Domineering decision-making

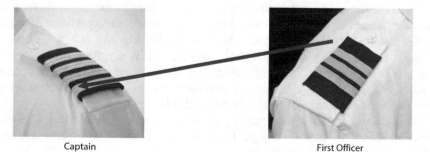

Captain   First Officer
TAG4. Reverse gradient. Very dangerous.

▣ **Fig. 8.4** An overview of possible authority gradients between the Captain and First Officer. An "authority gradient" refers to the official or perceived balance of power between a leader and his or her crew members. Credit: Authors

not otherwise meet expectations of their cockpit crewmembers. The machismo that previously defined "the right stuff" is no longer a desirable trait in commercial aviation—at least, not in such high doses.

Attitudes in general reflect people's ways of thinking or feeling about something—their likes and dislikes. Attitudes are reflected as a learned and lasting tendency for an individual to behave in a certain way. They have their roots in early life experiences and are generally affected by our environment. According to Hawkins [4], attitudes are said to have three components. The first is the *cognitive* component: the idea or knowledge about the object of the attitude. Second is the *affective* component: the feelings one holds about the object of the attitude. And lastly, the *behavioural* component: what the person says or does about it. In a flying scenario where a pilot might have an attitude regarding turbulence, the cognitive aspect is that the pilot knows about the effects of turbulence, the affective aspect is that the pilot does not like turbulence because it's uncomfortable and the passengers will complain, and the behavioural aspect is that the pilot avoids bad weather whenever possible to decrease the chance of encountering turbulence.

Many attitudes are based on stereotyping. We sometimes make incorrect assumptions about people based on their dress, the car they drive, their hairstyle, hair color, body piercings and tattoos. Stereotypes can have favorable or unfavorable associations. For example, we may be quick to discount the young-looking captain who settles into the left seat and defer to the gray-haired, more experienced-looking first officer settling into the right seat.

An issue studied by psychologists for years is the influence of groups on people's attitudes and behaviors. We all become members of groups over the course of our lives. Sports teams, fraternities, airlines, clubs, military branches, professional groups and even gangs draw people with a desire to join. In general, group members share many of the same values and goals, though not all. The desire to join a group is often made with the belief that the views of the group's members match one's own. In a person's need to belong, it is possible for group members to influence individuals into doing things they would not normally do. Taking risks seems more acceptable when done as part of a group. Shared blame or spreading out responsibility may make some previously unacceptable activities seem less risky.

Communication is key to modifying people's attitudes. Being an expert at persuasive communication is a skill those in the aviation business would do well to master. Persuasion is the act of convincing, inducing or enticing someone to do or believe something. The news of late has carried cellphone video of passengers being dragged off aircraft, resisting efforts to have them leave peacefully, whether due to overbooking, onboard pet issues or a host of other unpleasant reasons. Persuading passengers to stay calm in such conditions to keep the situation from escalating is important, though cabin personnel often find themselves in a contentious two-way debate, with each side trying to persuade the other as to what the outcome should be.

Persuasive communication regarding safety is somewhat paradoxical. One would think that receiving a message designed to save your life would be the easiest to accept and would have all passengers' undivided attention, but the before-takeoff safety briefing (◻ Fig. 8.5) largely continues to fall on deaf ears. According to safety experts, those who listen to the safety briefing and read the safety briefing cards do have a higher

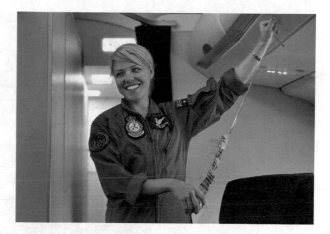

◘ Fig. 8.5 Royal Australian Air Force Leading Aircraftswoman Adele Taylor gives a safety brief to passengers on board the KC-30A Multi Role Tanker Transport before a flight in support of Cope North 13 on Anderson Air Force Base, Guam. Credit: USAF/Senior Airman Matthew Bruch

chance of survival. Attitudes toward safety must be established gradually [5]. Cautionary messages regarding the inherent risks in flying do not seem to be effective, though news of injuries during unexpected turbulence does seem to improve passengers' use of seat-belts during flight. Still, passengers will sometimes try to carry their rollaboard suitcases when evacuating an aircraft on fire.

8.1.5 Flight Training and Simulation

The path to the commercial cockpit has lengthened considerably in the past several years in the US. What once took only 250 flying hours now entails earning an Airline Transport Pilot (ATP) certificate requiring a minimum of 1,500 flying hours (with some options for restricted ATP qualifications). To achieve all requirements for the ATP, flight training may begin with private lessons with a Certified Flight Instructor without a specific syllabus, so long as all experience requirements for each certificate are met, or they can be taken at a flight school with an accredited syllabus. Generally, training consists of both Ground School and Flight Lessons.

A formal Ground School course is traditionally given as a lecture in a classroom by a Flight Instructor. Facilities and training aids specifically designed for pilot instruction are available, as well as other programmed instructional materials to supplement classroom instruction. Aeronautical theory is taught commensurate with the flight course the student is taking.

Flight lessons begin on the ground, though many students have experienced at least a 'Discovery Flight' to introduce them to flying. Afterward, the first real experience many aspiring pilots have before actually learning to fly is through simulation in a Cockpit Procedures Trainer (CPT) (◘ Fig. 8.6). These simulated cockpits are used to practice the most basic cockpit procedures, such as cockpit familiarization, preflight checklists and emergency procedures. Most or all systems and switches and knobs may be simulated. A CPT is typically very basic. After learning these basics, student pilots move on to flight, which is often done in conjunction with more simulator practice.

◘ Fig. 8.6 Cockpit procedures provide a useful platform for helping pilots learn preflight checklists and emergency procedures. Credit: Darren Sugden

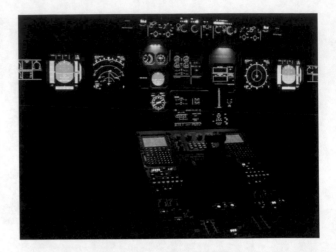

8

◘ Fig. 8.7 Full Flight Simulators provide motion simulation and in many cases are so realistic that it is possible for pilots to gain type ratings. Credit: Super Jet International

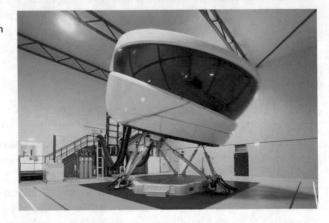

Aviation Training Devices (ATDs) are a step up from CPTs and are the most common option for general aviation (GA) flight training. Many flight schools use these devices to train their students as they prepare for private, instrument, multiengine and commercial pilot certificates. Depending on the features of the ATD, the FAA will authorize pilots to log some training hours toward proficiency requirements. ATDs have come a long way thanks to advancements in computers and other technology [6, 7].

The next step up is the Flight Training Device (FTD). This level of simulation represents specific aircraft conformations and often includes an enclosed cockpit and even realistic visual representations in the cockpit windows. While not usually capable of motion, they do provide a level of sophistication that makes them more representative of an actual aircraft, often with an enclosed cockpit area and more accurate visual references. FTDs are commonly used at aviation-centric universities and also by airlines training new-hire pilots, upgrading pilots from one seat to another, and for transitioning pilots from one type aircraft to another (B-757 to B-777).

Finally, a Full Flight Simulator (FFS) (pictured in ◘ Fig. 8.7) is a replica of an aircraft cockpit with the added benefit of motion. An FFS can represent both ground and flight

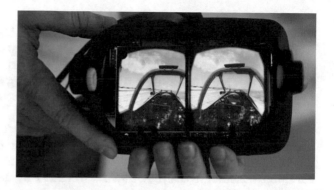

Fig. 8.8 Embry-Riddle Aeronautical University has some of the latest and greatest simulation devices, such as virtual reality. Credit: ERAU

conditions and operations and also provides a simulated outside view, meeting FAA performance standards for the level qualified. The costliest of all simulators, it is possible to earn aircraft type ratings in some of the more FFS advanced simulators without flying the actual aircraft. Until recently, these simulators relied on electrohydraulic actuators to replicate the actual feel of flying. Today, designers use the same concepts, but the actuators are all-electric, allowing for less downtime for maintenance. Training in a simulator is far less costly than training in an actual aircraft—a benefit all airlines enjoy [8, 9].

A mention is certainly due to our military counterparts, who follow a different but similar path to aviation careers. In 2018, a pilot trainee arriving at United States Air Force Undergraduate Pilot Training can expect to spend one year in academics and flight training, to include approximately 80 flying hours training in the T-6 Texan II, and another 60 hours flying the T-1 Jayhawk. From there, initial copilot training for those who go on to fly aircraft such as the C-17A and KC-15R lasts approximately 3–4 months. Many military pilots go on to fly for commercial airlines after leaving active duty.

8.1.6 Training Enhancement Strategies

Advances in technology reshape the possibilities for training every day. For example, video games have led to innovations used for unmanned flight, even in wartime. The aviation industry has become an innovator, and with the rising costs of training, the industry is quick to embrace new technologies that might enhance learning, training and pilot currency.

Training in most science, technology, engineering and math (STEM) career fields has changed to match today's students, who have grown up immersed in technology from a young age. They learn differently. The same teaching methods that worked in the 1970s are not guaranteed to work for the younger generations. They embrace simulation, gaming and interaction; they're tech-savvy, and they can multitask. A curriculum focused on the student must evolve to be effective.

In the hallways of modern universities, such as Embry-Riddle Aeronautical University in Daytona Beach, FL, some of the newest training devices can be seen already in use by students (□ Fig. 8.8). A virtual reality lab allows students and researchers to explore, develop and test immersive simulation technologies for use in aviation and aerospace research learning. Flying an F/A-18 Hornet to an aerial refueling is more than fun and games. Augmented reality devices, such as Google Glass, can superimpose digital data on top of our view of reality. Other wearable technology, such as smart clothing and fitness trackers, can provide other useful data that might be useful during flight training, since a student's physical state can affect flight. Did they get enough sleep? Are they impaired or stressed? Optimizing training might include checking their physical status before going out to fly. Most people perform better when they're feeling their best.

Big Data might also impact the way we hire employees in the first place. With the massive amounts of data generated by people every day, it may be possible in the not too distant future to compare the attributes of applicant pilots to a company's top performers through predictive analytics. Big data will likely be able to customize training per employee.

8.2 Summary

Training in aviation is evolving. Though CPTs and moving simulators have been a staple of pilot training for many years, the promises of new technology will potentially change the way we choose pilot trainees. Still, the basics of understanding one another as humans, learning to work together through CRM training and to identify and counter threats is of paramount importance.

Key Terms
ATC - Air Traffic Control
ATD - Aviation Training Device
ATP - Airline Transport Pilot
CPT - Cockpit Procedures Trainer
CRM - Crew Resource Management
FFS - Full Flight Simulator
FTD - Flight Training Device
GA - General Aviation
IATA - International Air Transport Association

Review Questions
1. What are positive and negative transfer?
2. What are internal and external threats?
3. What is CRM?
4. Describe the optimal transcockpit authority gradient
5. What are the three components of attitudes?
6. Why is it important to listen to the before-takeoff safety briefing?
7. What is the benefit of using a simulator for training versus flying an actual aircraft?
8. Give an example of new technology that might change the way we train people

References

1. Wise, J.A., Hopkin, V.D., Garland, D.J.: Handbook of Aviation Human Factors, 2nd edn. Taylor & Francis, Boca Raton (2010)
2. Cusick, S.K., Cortes, A.I., Rodrigues, C.C.: Commercial Aviation Safety, 7th edn. McGraw Hill, New York (2017)
3. Orlady, H.W., Orlady, L.: Human Factors in Multi-Crew Flight Operations. Ashgate, Cambridge (2017)
4. Hawkins, F.H.: Human Factors in Flight, 2nd edn. Ashgate, Burlington (1987)
5. Northedge, C., Anderson, R.: How to improve your chances of surviving a plane crash. The Guardian (U.S. Edition). Retrieved from https://www.theguardian.com/world/2009/feb/25/plane-crash-survival-tips (2009, Feb 25)
6. EUROCONTROL European Organisation for the Safety of Air Navigation: Proceedings of the Second EUROCONTROL Human Factors Workshop: Teamwork in Air Traffic Services. Retrieved from https://www.eurocontrol.int/sites/default/files/content/documents/nm/safety/safety-proceedings-of-the-second-eurocontrol-human-factors-workshop-1998.pdf (1998)
7. Bernard, M.: Real learning through flight simulation: the ABCs of ATDs. FAA Safety Briefing, 8–10. Retrieved from https://www.faa.gov/news/safety_briefing/2012/media/SepOct2012ATD.pdf (2012, Sept/Oct)
8. Bartel, C.: Flight simulators go from hydraulics to all-electric. Machine Design. Retrieved from https://www.machinedesign.com/motion-control/flight-simulators-go-hydraulics-all-electric (2014, June 9)
9. Kearns, S.: The future of technology in aviation training. Retrieved from the Uniting Aviation website: https://www.unitingaviation.com/strategic-objective/capacity-efficiency/the-future-of-technology-in-aviation-training/ (2017, Aug 11)

Suggested Reading

Northedge, C., Anderson, R.: How to improve your chances of surviving a plane crash. The Guardian (U.S. Edition). Retrieved from https://www.theguardian.com/world/2009/feb/25/plane-crash-survival-tips (2009, Feb 25)
Secretary of Aviation Report on Tenerife Crash: KLM, B-747, PH-BUF and Pan Am B-747 N736 collision at Tenerife Airport Spain on 27 March 1977. Retrieved from http://www.aviationcrin.com/TENERIFE.htm (1978)

Displays

© Springer Nature Switzerland AG 2020
E. Seedhouse et al., *Human Factors in Air Transport*,
https://doi.org/10.1007/978-3-030-13848-6_9

Learning Objectives

After completing this chapter, you should be able to

- Describe the primary functions of an electronic flight display
- List the key features of a multifunction display
- Explain how a heads-up display works
- List the key disadvantages and advantages of heads-up displays
- List the pros and cons of multifunction displays
- Explain how airborne collision avoidance systems work
- List the key elements of an enhanced vision system
- Distinguish between the three types of ACAS
- Explain how ACAS II works
- List the seven modes of a warning and advisory system

9

9.1 Introduction

Today, everyone is familiar with the glass cockpit, an evolution in aircraft human factors that originated in military aircraft in the late 1960s. Before the advent of the glass cockpit, aircraft displays relied on analog gauges. Some cockpits featured more than one hundred cockpit instruments and controls, which meant cockpit elements competed for cockpit space and pilot attention. As aircraft complexity increased and as air traffic congestion grew, so did the requirement for a more integrated flight system. This prompted NASA to conduct research on displays that could better present the flight situation; hence the glass cockpit was born.

During the 1970s, the glass cockpit gradually became more accepted, with the result that safety and flight efficiency increased, thanks in part to the way in which this type of flight display enhanced a pilot's situational awareness [1]. Glass cockpits quickly became standard on airliners, business jets and even the Space Shuttle (◘ Fig. 9.1). And, as the technology was scaled down and made more affordable, the glass cockpit began to appear in general aviation aircraft by the mid-2000s. In 2003, the Cirrus SR22 (◘ Fig. 9.2)

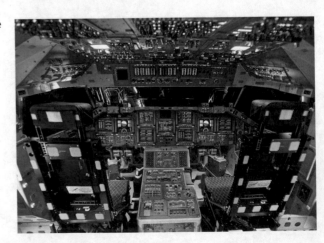

◘ **Fig. 9.1** Cockpit of the Space Shuttle Endeavor. Credit: NASA

9.2 · Electronic Flight Display

Fig. 9.2 2003–2008 era Cirrus instrument panel with the Avidyne Entegra primary flight display. Credit: Vectorstofinal

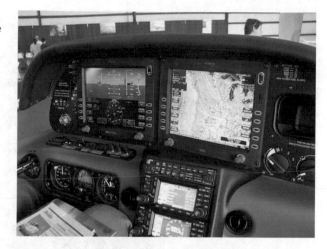

Fig. 9.3 EFIS on an Airbus A380. Credit: CC-BY-2.0

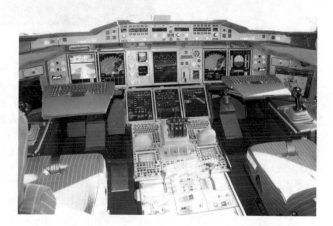

became the first GA aircraft to be equipped with a glass cockpit. Cessna, Piper and Diamond quickly followed suit. At the time of writing, the latest evolution in operational cockpit display technology can be seen in the F-35, which sports a panoramic cockpit display touchscreen system that has done away with almost all switches and toggles found in more conventional aircraft.

9.2 Electronic Flight Display

Today's instrument flight display is known as the electronic flight instrument display, or EFIS. The EFIS (■ Fig. 9.3) displays flight data electronically, whereas before this data was displayed electromechanically. The EFIS comprises of a primary flight display (PFD), a multi-function display (MFD) and an engine indicating and crew alerting system (EICAS) display. We'll take a look at each of these separately in the following section.

9

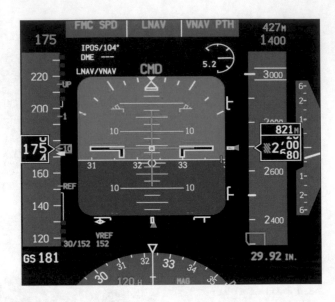

9.2.1 Primary Flight Display

The key elements of the PFD (□ Fig. 9.4) are those that give this display the appearance of a so-called *glass cockpit*. This display provides the pilot with all flight-critical data, including airspeed, altitude, heading and vertical speed. Since all this data is grouped together on a single display rather than separate instruments (as was the case in the 1970s), the pilot doesn't have to spend valuable time scanning. Instead, all it takes is a quick glance at the PFD. Thanks to the PFD, situational awareness is increased dramatically. There are variations in PFD design. For example, some PFDs will use two separate screens to show flight data and navigation, whereas others will combine this information on one PFD [2].

9.2.2 Engine Indication and Crew Alerting System

The EICAS is a system dedicated to displaying data about aircraft systems. Some of these displays echo the design of the old electromechanical gauges, since information is displayed on round gauges. For the most part, a lot of the data is presented in graphical format, which allows the pilot to process complex information quickly. The EICAS is also fitted with various alerts for thresholds such as oil pressure, exhaust gas temperature, hydraulic pressure and engine vibration.

9.2.3 Human Factors

9.2.3.1 Clutter

While all this advanced instrumentation can make the life of a pilot a lot less stressful, there are a number of human factors that can conspire to do the opposite. For example, during the different flight phases the pilot needs to access different groups of data

▣ Table 9.1	Color schemes used in EFIS displays
Green	Active or selected mode and/or dynamic conditions
White	Status situation and scales
Magenta	Command information, pointers, symbols and fly to tracks. Also used on weather radar to indicate possible turbulence
Cyan	Non-active and background information
Red	Warnings
Yellow/Amber	Cautions, flags and faults
Black	Blank areas or system off

specific to those phases. That means that the data that the pilot doesn't need doesn't have to be presented: if it is presented on the display, it becomes clutter, which distracts the pilots and reduces their SA. One example would be the glide slope indicator—the pilot doesn't need this when the aircraft is cruising at 35,000 feet, so the GSI is superfluous in the cruise phase of flight. Another example is engine vibration. This particular item does not need to be displayed at any phase of flight, but if parameters are exceeded then the pilot needs to be alerted. To help pilots make sense of valid and erroneous data, the EFIS is designed with a de-clutter mode that performs automatically. This de-clutter mode helps pilots focus on the most important tasks and thereby increases SA [3].

9.2.3.2 Color

The older electromechanical instruments used color but lacked the function of changing color to indicate a change in status. The EFIS does not have this drawback. Having said that, too many colors indicating different types of data can be confusing, which is why EFIS displays use standard color schemes as indicated in ▣ Table 9.1.

9.3 Multifunction Displays

The MFD displays navigation and weather data to the pilot. The most common MFD design is a chart-centric one that allows the pilot to overlay different information onto a chart. For example, the pilot may want to overlay the route plan and weather information onto the chart. Or perhaps the pilot would like to display information about aircraft systems.

The first multifunction displays (MFD) appeared in military aircraft such as the F-111D in the late 1960s. The advantage of such a system is that it did away with the traditional analog displays that made the old cockpits (known as "steam" cockpits in the aviation industry at the time) seem cramped, clustered and downright claustrophobic in some cases due to the sheer number of mechanical gauges. This new generation of displays enabled pilots to access a whole range of information—moving map, weather radar, navigation route, traffic collision avoidance system—on just one screen. In short, MFDs simplified aircraft operation and allowed pilots to focus more on flying the aircraft rather than checking gauges. MFDs also helped eliminate the flight engineer, thereby saving costs.

As with any technology, MFDs have evolved, as can be seen in a comparison between the early glass cockpit of the Boeing 737 and the more recent Airbus A320. One way these displays have been improved over the years is by the introduction of more modern sensors. For example, gyroscopes have been replaced with attitude and heading reference systems and GPS receivers. Another improvement has been to completely replace the traditional gauges (which were retained until the late 1990s as a back-up system) with the digital system. More recent advances have included the use of a trackball and/or joystick as a pilot-input device and the inclusion of synthetic vision systems (SVS), which are discussed later.

9.3.1 Layout

The PFD must provide the pilot with a myriad of data—air pressure, airspeed, vertical speed, weather radar—and this data can be presented in varying degrees of appearance and functionality. How all this data is presented depends to a degree on the aircraft, the type of PFD and the aircraft's manufacturer. Having said that, most PFDs present data according to a conventional layout as follows:

- Attitude Indicator (AI). This instrument, which usually sits in the center of the console, provides the pilot with information about pitch and roll. It is designed to look almost identical to the traditional mechanical display. Additional information that can be presented on this display include stall angle, ILS localizer and glide path indicators.
- Airspeed and Altitude. The airspeed indicator shows the aircraft's speed in knots and the altitude indicator shows the altitude of the aircraft above mean sea level (AMSL). These indicators, which usually present information as vertical "tapes" that scroll up and down, are positioned either side of the AI. Additional information that may be presented on these indicators includes "bugs" such as V speeds, do-not-exceed speeds, stall speeds and important altitudes.
- Vertical Speed Indicator. This indicator is usually positioned next to the altitude indicator. It provides the pilot with the rate of ascent and rate of descent and also how fast the aircraft is ascending or descending. This information is usually displayed in thousands of feet per minute.
- Heading Display. This display provides the pilot with rate of turn, current track (the path over the ground), current heading and the magnetic heading of the aircraft.
- Additional Data. The above data represents the minimum layout of a PFD. Additional displays may include course deviation indicators, ILS glideslope indicators and autopilots. We'll discuss some of these later in this chapter.

9.3.2 Pros and Cons

Due to the variability in PFD layout, pilots must be wary of the differences between aircraft types. Although the basic flight information is very similar across aircraft types, supplementary information such as angle of attack may be presented a number of ways using different graphics. Another consideration is failure of the system. Early in the operation of

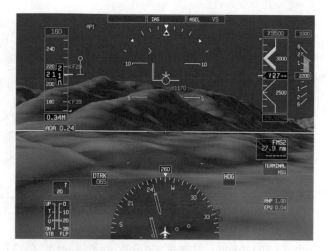

Fig. 9.5 A modern synthetic vision system produced by Honeywell. Credit: Honeywell

the Airbus A320, the company reported more than 50 incidents in which multiple displays malfunctioned. On January 25, 2008, United Airlines Flight 731 lost radio contact and half of the flight displays. So, while the use of PFDs has generally made flying safer and reduced workload, the technology has proved less than robust early in its adoption.

9.4 Synthetic Vision System

After many years of research, the NASA-developed synthetic vision system (SVS) first saw the light of day in 2005 when a system was installed on a Gulfstream V test aircraft. After a few more years of testing, the FAA certified the system in 2009. At its core, SVS is a system that uses three-dimensional data to provide intuitive displays that help increase the pilot's situational awareness (SA) regardless of weather conditions or visibility. By enhancing SA, SVS reduces pilot workload, especially during operationally demanding phases of flight such as approaches. The way the SVS (**Fig. 9.5**) achieves this is through a fusion of data (terrain database, data feed from nearby aircraft, obstacle data) that provides the pilot with a high-fidelity model of the real world in a way that is easily accessible and, most importantly, quickly understood [4].

One way SVS is used by showing a Highway in the Sky that depicts the projected flight path. This particular mode does a great job of enhancing a pilot's SA by utilizing myriad databases containing information about terrain, obstacles, hydrological and other environmental features. The system then fuses this information by means of an image generator computer and the display itself.

9.5 Enhanced Vision System

A close technological cousin of SVS, enhanced vision systems (EVS) utilize data from aircraft-based sensors such as infrared cameras to provide pilots with enhanced vision in limited visibility environments (haze, fog, night). EVS technology such as night vision systems have been available to military pilots for several years, but as the technology was

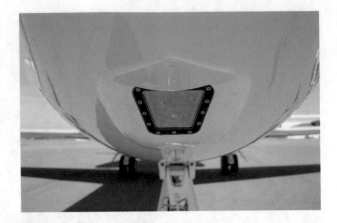

◘ Fig. 9.6 The forward-facing camera used for the PlaneView EVS on a Gulfstream G450. Credit: Spartan7W

refined and became more affordable, the general aviation industry began to incorporate the enhanced vision capabilities, with business jets the first adopters: in 2003, Gulfstream Aerospace offered IR as standard equipment on their Gulfstream G550. Six years later, the business jet company had delivered more than 500 aircraft equipped with EVS. Once business aviation began applying EVS technology, it wasn't long before the rest of the commercial aviation world followed suit, with Boeing offering EVS on the B787.

The great advantage of EVS is that safety is increased for almost all flight phases, but *especially* during approach and landing. Thanks to the enhanced vision, a pilot is able to make sense of the runway environment much earlier in the preparations for landing. That's because obstacles such as buildings, other aircraft on the runway, and terrain that might not be as clearly visible without the use of EVS are clear as day when using enhanced vision technology. Adding this extra layer of safety has prompted the FAA to grant revised operating minimums for aircraft equipped with EVS. What this means is that those aircraft with EVS (◘ Fig. 9.6) can fly a Category I approach in Category II minimum conditions. This change in regulations is a boon for aircraft operators, airports and passengers. Why? Well, if an aircraft is not equipped with EVS, it will not be permitted to descend to low altitude in low visibility to spot the runway. Instead, the non-EVS aircraft will be required to perform a missed approach and be sent on its way to another airport.

9.6   Warning And Advisory

9.6.1   Ground Proximity and Warning System

For a pilot flying at 20,000 feet, a 22,000-foot mountain looming directly ahead can make for a bad day. A really bad day. Crashing an aircraft into a mountain—or any part of the landscape—is an act that has its own acronym: Controlled Flight into Terrain (CFIT). Before the invention of Ground Proximity and Warning Systems (GPWS), also known (in the US) as a Terrain Awareness Warning System (TAWS), the rate at which aircraft crashed into terrain was two per year in the mid-1970s. That figure dropped following a FAA 1974 requirement that made it compulsory for all large aircraft to carry a GPWS.

More advanced versions of these systems, which were introduced in the late 1990s, are known as Enhanced Ground Proximity Warning Systems (EGPWS). These systems, which have the ability to look ahead and downwards, rely on GPS data to determine the aircraft's position, ground track and ground speed. All this information is processed by an onboard computer, which has a database containing information about all the world's natural terrain and manmade obstacles. The visual representations of this information are rendered on the screen, and the aircraft's position and flight path is superimposed onto that visual representation. The result is that the pilot is forewarned of any potential dangers via visual and aural warnings. If the pilot begins to fly towards any terrain, a warning sounds a minute prior to impact. Most EGPWS emit the following alarms:

- MODE 1. Excessive descent rate during landing.
- In this case the pilot receives the aural warning "Sink rate". If the pilot ignores the warning, the next aural warning is "Pull up".
- MODE 2. Excessive Terrain Closure Rate.
- If the aircraft is flying into a mountain (or ground clearance is decreasing quickly), the pilot will hear the warning "Terrain". This will quickly be followed by the enunciation "Pull up".
- MODE 3. Altitude Loss after Takeoff
- This mode is designed to help the pilot maintain a positive climb following takeoff. If after reaching 1,000 feet the aircraft begins to lose altitude, the enunciation "Don't sink" is broadcast.
- MODE 4. Unsafe Terrain Clearance
- This mode warns the pilot that the landing gear or flaps are in the incorrect configuration for landing by enunciating the following: "Too Low—Terrain", or "Too Low—Gear", or "Too Low—Flaps".
- MODE 5. Excessive Deviation below Glideslope
- If, when approaching the runway the aircraft deviates from the ILS approach, this mode warning enunciates "Glide slope".
- MODE 6. Excessively Steep Bank Angle
- The enunciation for this configuration is simply "Bank Angle".
- MODE 7. Windshear Protection.
- "Windshear".

» CFIT ("controlled flight into terrain") occurs when an airworthy aircraft is flown, under the control of a qualified pilot, into terrain (water or obstacles) with inadequate awareness on the part of the pilot of the impending collision.

- FAA definition of CFIT

9.6.2 Military GPWS Systems

For fighter jets, the use of mainstream GPWS systems isn't really practical because of the speed and low altitude at which this category of aircraft flies. To take into account these flying variables, an enhanced system is used that processes inputs from the radar altimeter, the inertial navigation system, GPS and the flight control system. By using data

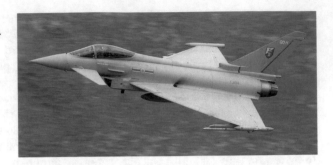

Fig. 9.7   Royal Air Force Eurofighter EF-2000 Typhoon F2. Credit: RAF

feeds from these systems, the military versions of GPWS (known as Automatic Ground Collision Avoidance System or Auto-GCAS; see Aside) can predict the flight path up to 8 km ahead. Such a system is standard onboard the Eurofighter Typhoon (Fig. 9.7).

Aside

May 5, 2016

A student was undergoing basic fighter training with his instructor in two F-16s. The student performed a roll maneuver and began to pull the aircraft, but the onset of Gs was too great and the student suffered a G-LOC (gravity-induced loss of conscious-ness) incident as the aircraft G-meter exceeded 8 G. This occurred at an altitude of 17,000 feet. The nose of the aircraft dropped and entered a dive—in full afterburner mode! 22 seconds later, the aircraft was nose-down and flying supersonic. As the F-16 plum-meted through 12,000 feet at a speed exceeding 580 knots, the instructor called "2 recover". Two seconds later the F-16 had steepened its dive to a 55° dive angle and had exceeded 600 knots. The instructor repeated the call. Two seconds later, he made the call a third time. At this stage, the F-16 was speeding along at 652 knots and had descended through 9,000 feet. Which is when the Auto-GCAS kicked in and saved the day.

» *My memory is that I started the fight and then I could see my instructor and the next thing I remember is just waking up. It feels weird because I think I'm waking up from my bed. In my helmet, I can hear him screaming 'recover, recover' at me and when I open my eyes I just see my legs and the whole cockpit. It doesn't really make sense. I got up over the horizon pretty fast again. It's all thanks to the Auto-GCAS system, which got me out of the roll and started the recovery for me. About maybe 30 seconds to a minute after I had gotten everything under control again. The first thing I thought about was my girlfriend, and then my family, and then my friends back home, and the thought of them basically getting a call [that I had perished]. This was an isolated incident for me, but, from the bottom of my heart, I just want to say thank you to everyone who has been a part of developing the Auto-GCAS system. It's everyone, not just engineers, but politicians and people just trying to get the ball rolling on having the Air Force use it. They are the reason that I am able to stand here today and talk about it. I'm able to continue to fly the F-16, and I'm able to go home and see my family again. So thank you, so much.*

- Student pilot recalling his close encounter with death onboard a F-16 equipped with Auto-GCAS. The event was the fourth "save" of an aircraft by the Auto-GCAS system since it was introduced by the USAF in 2014.

9

9.6.3 **Airborne Collision Avoidance System**

While the Auto-GCAS and GPWS systems are designed to prevent close encounters with terrain, the Airborne Collision Avoidance System (ACAS) is designed to reduce the risk of mid-air collisions or near mid-air collisions. There are three types of ACAS, as described in ◘ Box 9.1.

Box 9.1   Types of ACAS (Source: ICAO)

- **ACAS I** gives Traffic Advisories (TAs) but does not recommend any manoeuvres. The only implementation of the ACAS I concept is TCAS I. These equipments are limited to interoperability and interference issues with ACAS II.
- **ACAS II** gives Traffic Advisories (TAs) and Resolution Advisories (RAs) in the vertical sense (direction). ACAS II is the only commercially available implementation of the ICAO standard for this system. ACAS II is an aircraft system based on Secondary Surveillance Radar (SSR) transponder signals. ACAS II interrogates the Mode C and Mode S transponders of nearby aircraft and from the replies tracks their altitude and range and issues alerts to the pilots as appropriate. ACAS II works independently of the aircraft navigation, flight management systems and Air Traffic Control (ATC) ground systems.
- **ACAS III** gives TAs and RAs in vertical and/or horizontal directions. ICAO SARPs for ACAS III have not been developed.

The current system—ACAS II—is based on transponder signals emitted by secondary surveillance radar and interrogation of Mode C and Mode S transponders of nearby aircraft. ACAS II works separately from other aircraft navigation systems and air traffic control systems. It also works independently of the aircrafts autopilot. ACAS II can issue two types of alert, one being the Traffic Advisory (TA) and the other the Resolution Advisory (RA), which assists the pilot in visually acquiring an aircraft that may be on a collision path. If ACAS II decides there is a risk of collision, the system will generate a RA. The RA provides the pilot with information about the vertical speed the aircraft should be flown to avoid the other aircraft. Once the risk of collision has passed, the ACAS II enunciates "Clear of Conflict". But the system doesn't work on just one aircraft. The threat aircraft's RA coordinates with the other aircraft via a Mode S link, which basically means two ACAS II systems talk to each other to enable the pilots to select avoidance maneuvers. The target of the RAs is to establish a vertical separation of at least 300 feet. The timeline for a collision avoidance maneuver to occur is quite short. The TA may be generated less than a minute prior to Closest Point of Approach (CPA), and a RA may be generated in half that time [5] (◘ Fig. 9.8).

Each aircraft that is equipped with ACAS II is protected by a volume of airspace—a hazard or protection area—the size of which is determined by the size of the aircraft, the altitude it is flying, its speed and the heading of the aircraft. Armed with this information, the TCAS system generates a three dimensional map that is the protection area (◘ Fig. 9.9).

9

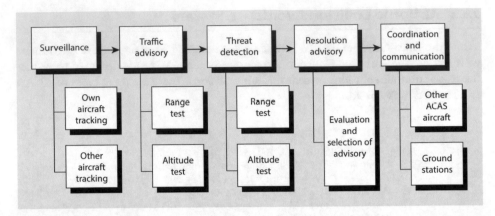

◻ Fig. 9.8   ACAS Functions. Source: ICAO Airborne Collisions Avoidance System Manual

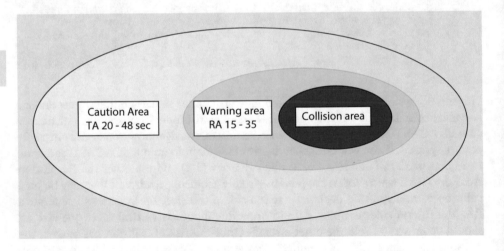

◻ Fig. 9.9   ACAS II Protection Area

9.6.4 **Complying with RAs**

If a RA is issued all pilots must comply, even if the RA contradicts an ATC clearance, unless by following the RA the pilot endangers another aircraft. By complying with the RA, the pilot will most likely deviate from the ATC clearance, at which point the controller has no responsibility for separation of the aircraft to which the RA was issued. Some examples are provided in ◻ Table 9.2 below.

Audio	Meaning	Required action
Climb, climb	Intruder will pass below	Begin climbing at 1,500–2,000 feet/min
Descend, descend	Intruder will pass above	Begin descending at 1,500–2,000 feet/min
Adjust vertical speed, adjust	Intruder is probably well above or below	Descend or climb at a slower rate
Maintain vertical speed, maintain	Intruder will be avoided if vertical rate is maintained	Maintain current vertical rate
Crossing	Passing through the intruder's level. Usually added to any other RA	Proceed according to the associated RA
Level off, level off	Intruder is no longer a threat while maintaining this level	Maintain current level (no climb, no descent)

◘ Table 9.2 Examples of RAs

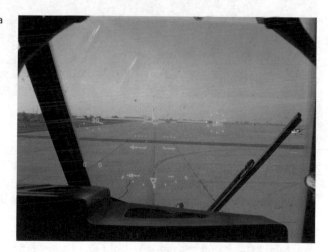

◘ **Fig. 9.10** Co-pilot's HUD of a C-130J. Credit: USAF

9.6.5 Heads-Up Display

» The beauty of a HUD is that it gets the pilot's eyes outside the cockpit and keeps them there. There's no need to constantly look up and look down and divide your attention between the instrument panel and the outside world. You get all the information you want while looking outside.

- Chuck Nash, a former US Navy pilot, who developed the non-TSO HUD

Head-up displays (◘ Fig. 9.10), or HUDs. You've all seen them, but what are they? Very simply, a HUD (Aside) presents information to the pilot in line with the pilots' forward vision by projecting flight data onto a small transparent screen located just in front of the pilot's line of sight [6]. Thanks to collimators and holographic technology, the image the pilot sees appears to be in front of the aircraft, which means the pilot does not have to change focus to see the data presented on the screen, which is usually about eight inches away from the pilot's eye.

» I could put a bullet through the window of a moving truck two miles away with a HUD because they allow you to fly so precisely. For GA pilots flying instrument approaches, the biggest advantage is that they can "see" the runway while they're still in the clouds. The transition from flying on the gauges and then switching to visual references also gets minimized because you're looking outside throughout the entire approach and landing.

- Steve Jacobson, an Avidyne executive and former US Air Force A–10 pilot

---

Aside

HUD in a Nutshell

A HUD system comprises the following elements:

— A computer that receives data from the aircraft and generates the display
— The overhead unit that projects the images onto the transparent display screen in front of the pilot.
— A transparent display—the *combiner* in HUD parlance—which is a holographic optical element. The combiner reflects the projected image to the pilot's eyes.
— A control panel that allows the pilot to select display options and to enter any information that is not integrated by the computer
— An enunciator panel that provides HUD status

9.6.5.1 HUD Data

A HUD presents all the data needed to fly the aircraft. At a minimum, the most basic HUD will present airspeed, localizer, glideslope, altitude, flight-path marker, airspeed trend, angle-of-attack and runway depiction. More advanced systems will provide landing-flare cues, unusual attitude, runway distance remaining and TCAS advisories.

9.6.5.2 Advantages and Disadvantages

You might think that such an advanced display system is the solution to all the issues that must be tackled when using conventional displays, and for the most part you would be correct. But, there are still a few problems. For example, HUDs can induce attention capture, a phenomenon also known as tunneling. When this occurs, the pilot becomes so fixated on the HUD display that some external cues may be excluded. Another problem is clutter, which may occur when outside cues may be obscured by display images.

For the most part, HUDs are a boon to pilots for a number of reasons. One benefit of a HUD system is the increase in situational awareness (SA) that is afforded to the pilot. This enhancement in SA is achieved because the pilot can sustain a constant external lookout without having to break their outside scan by glancing down at the instrumentation panel. This benefit is particularly advantageous during the takeoff, approach and landing phases of flight, which are when the majority of accidents occur.

9.7 Summary

In this chapter we reviewed the evolution of the glass cockpit and aircraft human factors that resulted in the cockpit of today. We also discussed how this evolution enhanced situational awareness and how the trend in reducing the number of switches and toggles has transformed the modern cockpit into a panoramic display touchscreen system. Additionally, we reviewed the various information metrics that are presented via a HUD, such as airspeed, localizer, glideslope, altitude, flight-path marker, airspeed trend, angle-of-attack and runway depiction.

Key Terms

ACAS - Airborne Collision Avoidance System

AI - Attitude Indicator

ATC - Air Traffic Control

CFIT - Controlled Flight into Terrain

CPA - Closest Point of Approach

EFIS - Electronic Flight Information Systems

EGPWS - Enhanced Ground Proximity Warning System

EICAS - Engine Indication and Crew Alerting System

EVS - Enhanced Vision System

G-LOC - Gravity-Induced Loss of Consciousness

GPWS - Ground Proximity Warning System

GSI - Ground Slope Indicator

HUD - Heads-Up Display

MFD - Multifunction Display

PFD - Primary Flight Display

SA - Situational Awareness

SVS - Synthetic Vision Display

TA - Traffic Advisory

TAWS - Terrain Awareness Warning System

Review Questions

1. What do the colors white, cyan and red denote in an EFIS?
2. List two advantages and two disadvantages of a PFD
3. What does Mode 2 denote in a TAWS?
4. What is the difference between an ACAS I and an ACAS II?
5. Which two types of alert can the ACAS II issue?
6. List two examples of Resolution Advisory
7. List two pros and two cons of a HUD
8. What is the combiner in a HUD?
9. What does Mode 5 denote in a TAWS?
10. What is the EICAS?

References

1. Shappell, S., Weigmann, D.: Reviewing the role of cockpit systems. In: Human Factors and Aerospace Safety, vol. 1 (nr. 1), pp. 59–86. Ashgate Publishing, Aldershot (2001)
2. Newman, R., Greeley, K.: Cockpit Display: Test and Evaluation. Ashgate Publishing Limited, Aldershot (2001)
3. CAA, P-NPA 25–310, Issue 1 Human Centered Design Requirements, Dated April 2000, Gatwick, UK (2000)
4. FAA: Human Factors Study Team Report on the Interface Between Flight Crews and Modern Flight Deck Systems. Federal Aviation Administration, Washington, DC (1996)
5. Rignèr, J., Dekker, S.: Modern flight training – managing automation or learning to fly? In: Dekker, S.W.A., Hollnagel, E. (eds.) Coping with Computers in the Cockpit, pp. 145–151. Ashgate, Hants (1999)
6. Wickens, C.: Attentional issues in head up displays. In: Harris, D. (ed.) Engineering Psychology and Cognitive Ergonomics, vol. 1, pp. 3–22. Ashgate, Aldershot (1997)

Suggested Reading by Topic

DO-315B Minimum Aviation System Performance Standards (MASPS) for Enhanced Vision Systems, Synthetic Vision Systems, Combined Vision Systems and Enhanced Flight Vision Systems, EUROCAE (Dec 2008)

FAA Advisory Circular No 20-167A: Airworthiness Approval of Enhanced Vision System, Synthetic Vision System, Combined Vision System, and Enhanced Flight Vision System Equipment (Dec 2016)

9

Flight Crew System-Based Training

© Springer Nature Switzerland AG 2020
E. Seedhouse et al., *Human Factors in Air Transport*,
https://doi.org/10.1007/978-3-030-13848-6_10

Learning Objectives

After completing this chapter, you should be able to

- Describe the rationale for competency-based training
- List the key features of CBT
- Explain how progression is assessed in the CBT process
- Explain what is meant by "lateral recruitment circumstances"
- Explain why virtual reality is helpful in training pilots
- List five advantages VR has over traditional learning
- Provide two examples of airlines using VR to train their personnel
- Explain what is meant by "augmented reality"
- Provide an example of how AR is used in the aviation industry

10.1 Introduction

In the discussion of human factors thus far, the common element in the majority of accidents has been the human. One reason for this can be traced to training. Human factors specialists have therefore sought to devise better ways to instruct pilots in the hope of reducing the accident rate. One such initiative is competency-based training, or CBT. CBT is a more holistic approach to learning, in which students are exposed to whole-task training. In CBT, interactivity is a key feature that endeavors to align activities with the training goal.

>> The key is to align the activity with a training goal and ensure it creates an authentic and realistic real-world scenario. When we were writing Competency-Based Education in Aviation, my coauthors and I had to interview several dozen aviation professionals from around the world to try and nail down a single definition. Also, the industry has some who are very strong advocates of CBT and others who are hesitant to adopt new approaches. The reality is that the concept has both strengths and limitations—the best implementation will be considerate of both. If you can't learn the way I teach, there are ten more people like you who can.

- Dr. Suzanne Kearns, coauthor of *Competency-Based Education in Aviation*

10.2 CBT in Aviation

Traditionally in aviation, a common practice by which to measure flight competency is flight hours. More flight hours equals more competence. Simple, right? It's a good metric, but one that doesn't consider quality of flight time or any practical experience gained by the pilot. For example, a pilot who has logged 3,000 hours flying a Cessna 172 in and around Toronto is not necessarily a more accomplished pilot than one who has logged 1,500 hours in eight aircraft types in a dozen locations. These metrics are important not only for pilot selection but for career progression from the right seat to the left seat. So what can airlines do? They can adopt CBT (◘ Fig. 10.1) by removing the prescriptive hour minimums and instead implementing a more structured approach based on competency. In this approach, the following metrics may be considered:

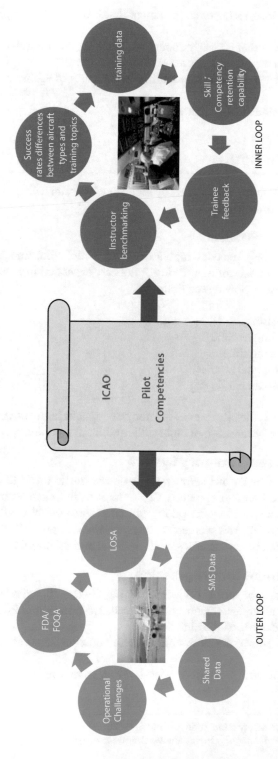

Fig. 10.1 Pilot competencies. Credit: ICAO

- Training for a license, rating or endorsement that is conducted to approved standards
- A training program that is clearly documented in a logical and relevant manner
- All results are correctly and comprehensively recorded
- Assessments that are rigorous, standardized and measured against approved standards
- Training that is validated by summative tests

10.2.1 CBT Framework

At its core, a CBT framework[1] adopted by an airline/operator will probably comprise the eight key elements outlined here.

10.2.1.1 Selection Process

This element most likely includes inputs from the Chief Pilot and the Director of Training. As part of the selection procedure, pilots are evaluated in a simulator and are required to possess the following requirements:

- Class 1 Medical
- 1,500 hours total time
- 500 hours multi-engine time
- 100 hours Command time
- Commercial Aeroplane License
- Multi-Engine Instrument Rating

In this element of CBT, the pilot is assessed not just on flight hours but also on an incremental and step-wise progression of flight skills and flight complexity.

10.2.1.2 Flight Crew Category System

The information used by the airline/operator to determine how a flight crew progresses in their career can be found in Appendix VII. At its core, this element stresses the competencies and skills acquired by the pilot/flight crew. For example, rather than simply checking boxes for skills, this element focuses on the demonstration of flying skills across a range of operational scenarios, both nominal and off nominal.

10.2.1.3 Assessment for Progression

To assess progression, the airline utilizes a training file that includes each progression stage together with all endorsements and approvals from the Chief Pilot. For example, such a file might include the following items:

- A syllabus that itemizes the aims, objectives and outcomes for each training element
- Minimum competencies required for each progression level

---

1   Adapted from Flight Safety International: Flight Crew Competency Based Training Framework: Fixed-Wing Transport Category Operations. Version 1, May 2015.

- Ground school training programs and examination requirements
- Airborne training programs and examination requirements
- Simulator training programs and examination requirements
- Category Upgrade checking forms
- Proficiency Check and Line Check forms

10.2.1.4 Use of Simulators

A full motion flight simulator combined with computer-based training (to familiarize pilots with flight management systems) is deemed a requirement for a CBT program, as are the following requirements:

- Line Oriented Flight Training (LOFT)
- Crew Resource Management (CRM)
- Airline's Simulator Flying Instructors/Examiners (SFI/SFEs)

10.2.1.5 Training and Checking Manual

This assessment criterion is most likely conducted by a Type Rating Instructor or Type Rating Examiner and follows the requirements outlined in the operators training manual. This criterion is essentially a standardization check.

10.2.1.6 Instrument and Night Flying

As with any aviation assessment procedure, instrument flying skills must be assessed and maintained. The CBT requirements for this are documented together with endorsements, and pilots are assessed on their ability to manage instrument modes of operation in normal and abnormal conditions.

10.2.1.7 Lateral Recruitment Circumstances

In the CBT scheme of assessment, these circumstances occur when a pilot's experience exceed those entry-level requirements outlined in the selection process. For example, a pilot may have significant multi-engine experience but little or no IFR experience. Or perhaps a pilot may have significant hours but little or no multi-crew experience. The CBT program can accommodate these circumstances by applying a personalized program to the individual's circumstances and experience.

10.2.1.8 Command

This element falls at the end of the CBT program and assesses the aptitude of a pilot to make Captain. To do that, the program incorporates the following elements:

- Ground training. This includes technical proficiency, aviation law, crew management, airmanship and situational awareness
- A Proficiency Check conducted in a simulator
- Line Checks conducted in the aircraft

The development of an industry-agreed CBT framework provides the catalyst for Operators to move away from the prescriptive approach historically used to recruit and promote flight crew to command positions. The incorporation of a robust CBT program will provide transparency into the operator's training regime and allow the necessary auditable assurance demanded by all clients of the industry.

10.3 **Virtual Reality**

The use of virtual reality (VR) is a natural evolution of computer-based training. Today this technology is available to anyone who has a smart phone, and this accessibility has resulted in myriad virtual learning environments (VLE) being designed for all sorts of applications [1, 2]. In these VLEs, the student can participate in the learning task with a sense of presence in a way that is not possible in formal education. Not surprisingly, VR has a number of advantages over traditional learning, namely by:

1. Providing new forms of visualization
2. Illustrating features and processes that permit close-up examination of objects
3. Motivating students to learn since VR requires interaction and encourages active participation
4. Allowing students to proceed through a learning experience at their own pace
5. Transcending language barriers
6. Allowing students to learn in contexts that are impossible in real life
7. Offering more personalized learning
8. Supporting new instructional approaches
9. Providing authentic and realistic scenarios
10. Enhancing real-life experience

VR can provide new experiences that enhance learning, but exactly how is it used in the world of aviation? The answer is pretty much everywhere. Think of all the trainers and simulators used in the aviation industry [3]. There are door trainers, cabin emergency evacuation trainers, over-wing exit trainers, cabin service trainers, evacuation slide towers, cockpit trainers, etc. The list goes on. Some of these trainers are very realistic, featuring tactile interaction using force feedback. But at the end of the day, crews need to experience real flight emotions. Consider all the aviation specialists involved in getting passengers from one city to another. The typical passenger may only interact with the flight attendant, but think about the customer service representatives, the flight dispatchers, ground crew technicians and the technicians. It's worth taking a look at how VR can be used to train these specialists.

10.3.1 **Preflight Inspection**

For those involved in training personnel involved in preflight, VR is a godsend. In fact, the technology is so effective that the International Air Transport Association (IATA) uses VR to train ground crew. Thanks to a head-mounted display (HMD, ◘ Fig. 10.2) and some nifty software, employees can virtually walk around any aircraft you care to mention and learn how to detect issues and conduct the myriad checks required to certify an aircraft for flight. In the real world, inspections are limited, but in the VR world it is possible to conjure up any scenario imaginable. For example, no company would intentionally damage an aircraft just to teach its personnel how to detect a particular issue, but in the immersive world of VR this is…well, easy. VR software developers can design any fuselage or wing defect you

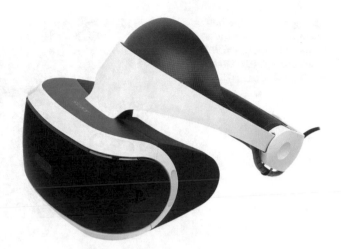

�‣ Fig. 10.2 The PlayStation VR, an example of a virtual reality head-mounted display for the Sony PlayStation 4 video game console. Credit: Evan-Amos

can think of and provide a learning experience that teaches ground crew to detect and resolve them. By doing that, VR can help ensure that crews are ready for any conceivable unexpected situation.

Additionally, VR takes place in a safe environment. Think about the world before VR. In that world, aviation engineers were unable to accumulate the practical experience that allowed them to resolve problems on complex equipment because they had to wait for it to become available. Not only that, but when the piece of complex equipment finally did become available, it was rarely possible for engineers to practice their skills in real situations. In VR, the equipment is available anytime and anywhere. Just plug in the HMD and away you go! It is for these reasons that Pratt and Whitney train their engineers and mechanics by using VR. In the Pratt and Whitney VR experience, engineers can inspect an engine, look inside, observe flow rates and do just about any conceivable procedure. Not only is such training safe and quick, but it also saves an inordinate amount of money.

10.3.2 **Crew Training**

Now let's take a look at how VR training can be applied to crew training (◘ Fig. 10.3). We'll begin with the flight attendants. These crewmembers must conduct a safety check to ensure that life-vests, flashlights and fire extinguishers are in working condition. They have to ensure no dangerous items enter the cabin, monitor the cabin for passenger behavior and perform the necessary safety demonstration. Before being certified as a flight attendant, these crewmembers must learn to deal with situations such as hijacking, water landings, critically ill passengers and water landings [4]. Until recently, this training was delivered via monotonous tutorials, endless PowerPoint presentations (yawn) and the occasional visit to an aircraft mock-up. Now, thanks to VR software such as aViatoR, airlines can accelerate flight attendant training and provide their staff with high-fidelity and realistic training environments. The outcome is a crew that is well-prepared for any situation the airline industry can throw at them.

◘ **Fig. 10.3**   Embry-Riddle Aeronautical University is pioneering the use of VR to train pilots. Credit: ERAU

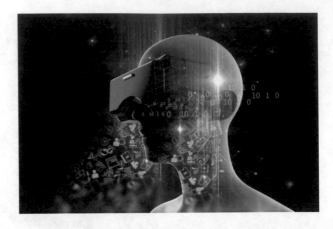

◘ **Fig. 10.4**   One way VR can be used is to provide safe immersive experiences of emergencies. Credit: US Marine Corps SSgt. Ricardo Morales, USMC

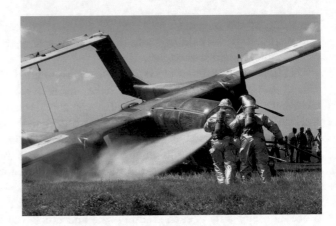

In the VR flight attendant world, trainees can interact within myriad cabin scenarios and become acquainted with the emotional condition they will face when presented with a contingency such as a passenger having a heart attack or a passenger threatening another with a knife.

10.3.3 **Flight Deck Training**

The flight crew must be trained in all sorts of tasks. Routine tasks are fairly easy to teach, but teaching someone how to deal with emergencies (◘ Fig. 10.4) demands more rigorous instruction. Once again, VR can help. Let's consider an example of just one dangerous situation: the electronic flight bag (EFB). As you know, the EFB is where pilots carry their tablets and other information management devices to perform flight management tasks. But what if there is a fire? If this happens, the pilot will place the EFB into a fire sock and extinguish the fire, but how to train pilots to do this? With a real fire? With VR, you can provide an immersive fire experience and safely train pilots in this task [5, 6].

10.3.4 Inflight Entertainment

As flights get longer and longer, inflight entertainment is assuming ever greater importance. With an Emirates flight from Dubai to Orlando taking more than 16 hours,
inflight entertainment is a must, which is why airlines such as Air France and Lufthansa
(Aside) have already adopted VR as part of their inflight entertainment. But the utility
of VR doesn't stop there. Ever been stressed out by screaming babies or other passengers
talking? VR offers a means to transport oneself to a completely different audiovisual
environment—Tahiti perhaps, or even the surface of Mars! Nothing is off limits.

》 VR is a growing trend for destination experiences and we wanted to help inspire our
passengers while they were in the sky. The Frankfurt to Dubai flight was a first-time
test for our new VR prototype, which was designed to further enhance the
passenger experience. I'm pleased to say this virtual exploration trip was very
positively received by the participating passengers.

- Paul Schön, Passenger Experience Designer for Lufthansa (interview with
▶ www.techradar.com, Aug 5, 2018)

Aside

How Airlines use VR and AR

Lufthansa uses VR as a means of enticing passengers to buy business class seats instead of economy class. The first Lufthansa passengers to experience this inflight entertainment were those flying from

Frankfurt to Dubai on Flight LH630 in 2018. Passengers were able to view the moving map in 3D and also experienced visual excursions. Meanwhile, Air France began trialing VR for its passengers in late 2017 in a partnership with SkyLights, while Air New Zealand uses Microsoft's HoloLens for its crew training.

》 These tasks are practiced to the point of mastery. Over-learned skills tend to be
maintained under stress because they have become automatic. So, over-learned
skills reduce the mental workload during a high-stress situation and improve the
odds of successfully executing the correct procedures. That's what makes the drilling
of those tasks so useful as preparation for an actual emergency.

- Dr. Chris Front, aerospace clinical psychologist, FAA Office of Aerospace Medicine

10.4 Augmented Reality

Another emerging technology closely related to VR is augmented reality (AR). What is
AR? When someone uses AR (◘ Fig. 10.5) they are presented with real-time information that is augmented by computer-generated perceptual information [7, 8]. For example, when a pilot is using AR when landing, perceptual information such as ATC, terrain
and airspace information may be overlaid on the actual perceptual information. Think
of a Heads-Up Display (HUD)—AR is very similar. Imagine when a pilot is navigating
to the runway for takeoff. In this application the AR system might present an overlay of

❏ **Fig. 10.5**   Google Glass is an example of an augmented reality platform that is being increasingly used in aviation training. Credit: Rijans007

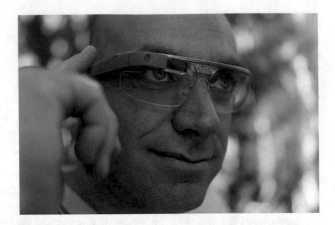

a corridor view to assist in navigating [9, 10]. And once the pilot is en-route, the AR system might present artificial horizons and terrain details to enhance situational awareness. AR can also be used to help train maintenance technicians, which is both a daunting and expensive process. But with AR, virtual images of components can be generated, resulting in an experiential learning environment that is safe and quick [11, 12]. Additionally, an AR environment can help pilots and flight personnel not only avoid costly mistakes but also make the right decisions in an immersive environment.

10

10.5 Summary

In this chapter we reviewed cutting-edge systems and displays in modern aircraft and how these have improved safety and resulted in a more economical operation of aircraft. We also discussed how a CBT framework provides the catalyst for airlines to move away from the prescriptive approach historically used to recruit and promote flight crew to command positions. Additionally, we reviewed how incorporating a robust CBT program can provide transparency into the operator's training regime and allow auditable assurance to be conducted by clients of the industry.

> **Key Terms**
> **AR** - Augmented Reality
> **CBT** - Competency-Based Training
> **CRM** - Crew Resource Management
> **EFB** - Electronic Flight Bag
> **HMD** - Head-Mounted Display
> **HUD** - Heads-Up Display
> **LOFT** - Line Oriented Flight Training
> **SFI** - Simulator Flight Instruction
> **VLE** - Virtual Learning Environment

Review Questions
1. What is the difference between VR and AR?
2. What is meant by competency-based training?
3. What is meant by "lateral recruitment process"?
4. List five advantages VR has over traditional learning
5. Describe two scenarios in which VR can be used for instruction

References

1. Gerbaud, S., Mollet, N., Arnaldi, B.: Virtual environments for training: from individual learning to collaboration with humanoids. Dans Edutainment. Retrieved from http://front.math.ucdavis.edu/0708.0712 (2007)
2. Bowman, D.A., Hodges, L.F., Allison, D., Wineman, J.: The Educational Value of an Information-Rich Virtual Environment (GVU Technical Report; GIT-GVU-98-05). Georgia Institute of Technology, Atlanta (1998)
3. Yavrucuk, I., Kubali, E., Tarimci, O.: A low cost flight simulator using virtual reality tools. IEEE Aerosp. Electron. Syst. Mag. **26**(4), 1014 (2011)
4. Duffy, V.G., Ng, P.P.W., Ramakrishnan, A.: Impact of simulated accident in virtual training on decision-making performance. Int. J. Ind. Ergon. **34**(4), 335–348 (2004)
5. Onyesolu, M.O., Eze, F.U.: Understanding Virtual Reality Technology: Advances and Applications. Virtual Reality. Intech Open (2009)
6. Lourdeaux, D., Fuchs, P., Burkhardt, J.-M.: An intelligent tutorial agent for training virtual environments. 5th World Multiconference on Systemics, Cybernetics and Informatics SCI'01. Orlando, FL (2001)
7. Dalgarno, B., Hedberg, J., Harper, B.: The contribution of 3D environments to conceptual understanding. In: Proceedings of the 19th Annual Conference of the Australian Society for Computers in Tertiary Education (ASCILITE). UNITEC Institute of Technology, Auckland (2002)
8. Ronald, A.T., Baillot, Y., Behringer, R., Feiner, S., Julier, S., MacIntyre, B.: Recent advances in augmented reality. IEEE Comput. Graph. Appl. **21**, 34–47 (2001)
9. Regenbrecht, H., Baratoff, G., Wilke, W.: Augmented reality projects in the automotive and aerospace industry. IEEE Comput. Graph. Appl. **25**(6), 48–56 (2005)
10. Foyle, D., Andre, A., Hooey, B.: Situation awareness in an augmented reality cockpit: design, viewpoints and cognitive glue. In: Proceedings of the 11th international conference on human computer interaction, Las Vegas, NV, USA. Available at http://hsi.arc.nasa.gov/groups/HCSL/publications/Foyle_HCI2005.pdf (2005)
11. Webel, S., Bockholt, U., Engelke, T., Gavish, B., Olbrich, M., Preusche, C.: An augmented reality training platform for assembly and maintenance skills. Robot. Auton. Syst. **61**, 398–403 (2013)
12. Hincapié, M., Caponio, A., Rios, H., Mendivil, E.G.: An introduction to Augmented Reality with applications in aeronautical maintenance 2011. In: 13th International Conference on Transparent Optical Networks, pp. 1–4 (2011)

Supplementary Information

© Springer Nature Switzerland AG 2020
E. Seedhouse et al., *Human Factors in Air Transport*,
https://doi.org/10.1007/978-3-030-13848-6

Appendices

Appendix I

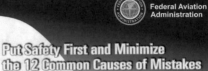

Federal Aviation
Administration

Avoid the
Dirty Dozen

Put Safety First and Minimize the 12 Common Causes of Mistakes in the Aviation Workplace

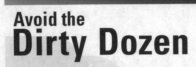

12 Common Causes of Human Factors Errors

About **80** Percent of Maintenance Mistakes Involve **Human Factors** ... and if Not Detected... Would Lead to Accidents.

① Lack of Communication
Failure to transmit, receive, or provide enough information to complete a task. Never assume anything.

Only 30% of verbal communication is received and understood by either side in a conversation. Others usually remember the first and last part of what you say.

Improve your communication—
- Say the most important things in the beginning and repeat them at the end.
- Use checklists.

② Complacency
Overconfidence from repeated experience performing a task.

Avoid the tendency to see what you expect to see—
- Expect to find errors.
- Don't sign it if you didn't do it.
- Use checklists.
- Learn from the mistakes of others.

③ Lack of Knowledge
Shortage of the training, information, and/or ability to successfully perform.

Don't guess, know—
- Use current manuals.
- Ask when you don't know.
- Participate in training.

 FAASTeam
FAA SAFETY TEAM   **www.FAASafety.gov**   YOUR SOURCE FOR AVIATION SAFETY

Avoid These Common Causes of Mistakes in the Aviation Workplace

Distractions
Anything that draws your attention away from the task at hand.

Distractions are the #1 cause of forgetting things, including what has or has not been done in a maintenance task.

Get back in the groove after a distraction—
- Use checklists.
- Go back 3 steps when restarting the work.

Lack of Teamwork
Failure to work together to complete a shared goal.

Build solid teamwork—
- Discuss how a task should be done.
- Make sure everyone understands and agrees.
- Trust your teammates.

Fatigue
Physical or mental exhaustion threatening work performance.

Eliminate fatigue-related performance issues—
- Watch for symptoms of fatigue in yourself and others.
- Have others check your work.

Lack of Resources
Not having enough people, equipment, documentation, time, parts, etc., to complete a task.

Improve supply and support—
- Order parts before they are required.
- Have a plan for pooling or loaning parts.

Pressure
Real or perceived forces demanding high-level job performance.

Reduce the burden of physical or mental distress—
- Communicate concerns.
- Ask for extra help.
- Put safety first.

Lack of Assertiveness
Failure to speak up or document concerns about instructions, orders, or the actions of others.

Express your feelings, opinions, beliefs, and needs in a positive, productive manner—
- Express concerns but offer positive solutions.
- Resolve one issue before addressing another.

Stress
A physical, chemical, or emotional factor that causes physical or mental tension.

Manage stress before it affects your work—
- Take a rational approach to problem solving.
- Take a short break when needed.
- Discuss the problem with someone who can help.

Lack of Awareness
Failure to recognize a situation, understand what it is, and predict the possible results.

See the whole picture—
- Make sure there are no conflicts with an existing repair or modifications.
- Fully understand the procedures needed to complete a task.

Norms
Expected, yet unwritten, rules of behavior.

Help maintain a positive environment with your good attitude and work habits—
- Existing norms don't make procedures right.
- Follow good safety procedures.
- Identify and eliminate negative norms.

Visit us at:
www.FAASafety.gov
Your Aviation Safety Web Site

Appendix II

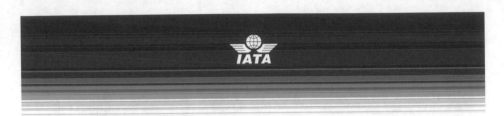

Fatigue Risk Management Systems (FRMS)

Introduction

In November 2011, the International Civil Aviation Organization (ICAO) released an amendment to Annex 6 *Operation of Aircraft*, Part 1, Section 4 Flight Operations and Appendix 8 FRMS Requirements. The amendment introduced a science-based approach to flight and duty time limitations (FTLs) and provided a framework for Regulators to facilitate regulation to oversee FRMS. Prior to this amendment, the only international standards available for managing fatigue in flight operations were related to prescriptive FTLs.

The traditional regulatory approach to manage crewmember fatigue has been to prescribe limits on maximum flight and duty hours, and required minimum breaks within and between duty periods. It is a one-size-fits-all approach that does not take into account operational differences. FRMS is an enhancement to FTLs, enabling an operator to customize FTLs to better manage fatigue risk to the operation. There is scientific and operational support that FRMS will become a means for effectively mitigating fatigue risks.

ICAO, IATA & IFALPA released an *FRMS Implementation Guide for Operators*[1] and ICAO an *FRMS Manual for Regulators*[2] which provide detailed information for Operators and Regulators on implementing FRMS.

All States are currently required to have prescriptive regulations (FTLs) for fatigue management. This requirement will continue whether or not they choose to implement regulations for an FRMS.

What is an FRMS?

ICAO defines an FRMS as *'A data-driven means of continuously monitoring and managing fatigue-related safety risks, based on scientific principles and knowledge as well as operational experience that aims to ensure relevant personnel are performing at adequate levels of alertness.'* (ICAO, 2011)

FRMS, by applying the Safety Management System (SMS) principles of risk identification, assessment, mitigation and monitoring, provides a performance-based approach to manage fatigue risk.

Like SMS, FRMS seeks to achieve a realistic balance between safety, productivity and cost.

---

[1] *FRMS Implementation Guide for Operators*, 1st Edition, July 2011, IATA, ICAO, IFALPA
[2] *FRMS Manual for Regulators*, ICAO Doc 9966, 2011 Edition

FRMS Principles

The FRMS Implementation Guide for Operators was a result of the combined efforts of ICAO, IATA & IFALPA, representing the three parties to FRMS; the regulator, the operator and the crewmember. Trust between all parties is vital to ensure the success of FRMS.

A key feature of FRMS is that responsibility for managing fatigue risk is shared between operators and individual crewmembers. For example, operators are responsible for providing rest opportunities while crewmembers have a responsibility to use rest periods effectively.

As in SMS, the FRMS relies on the concept of an "effective reporting culture" with active involvement of all stakeholders where personnel are constantly encouraged to report hazards whenever observed in the operational environment for the attainment of optimum safety levels and a continuous improvement program.

What are the benefits of FRMS?

Generic prescriptive regulations (FTLs) may not address operational peculiarities and complexities. FRMS policies and procedures focus on the operator's specific operations (e.g., continuous duty overnights, night versus day operations, short-haul versus long-haul, etc.). Therefore, an FRMS allows an operator to adapt policies, procedures and practices to the specific conditions that result in fatigue risk in a particular aviation setting. Operators may tailor their FRMS to meet their unique operational demands and focus on fatigue mitigation strategies that are specific to their operational environment.

In addition to fatigue mitigation, some of the benefits of an FRMS are:

- A reduction in fatigue related errors, incidents and accidents – which may be associated with financial costs and/or impact an operator's reputation.

- Reduced insurance costs – some insurers may reduce premiums if the operator can demonstrate that fatigue risk is being managed.

- Reduced absenteeism – operators may notice a decrease in sickness and other absences which were related to fatigue.

- Attracting and retaining crew – 'fatigue friendly' rosters may attract and retain crew as a result of an improved work/life balance. Fatigue at work is more effectively managed, increasing morale.

Summary

FRMS provides a performance-based regulatory approach which defines requirements for operators to manage fatigue risk, rather than only prescribing FTLs that may not consider aspects specific to the organization or operating environment.

Appendix III

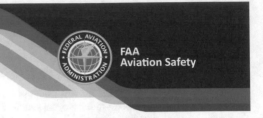

General Aviation
Joint Steering Committee
Safety Enhancement Topic

March 2015

FAA
Aviation Safety

Single-Pilot Crew Resource Management

There is no one right answer in aeronautical decision-making. Each pilot is expected to analyze each situation in light of experience level, personal minimums, and current physical and mental readiness level, and make his or her own decision.

Single-pilot resource management (SRM) is the art of managing all onboard and outside resources available to a pilot before and during a flight to help ensure a safe and successful outcome. Incorporating SRM into GA pilot training is an important step forward in aviation safety. A structured approach to SRM helps pilots learn to gather information, analyze it, and make sound decisions on the conduct of the flight.

5P Approach to SRM

To get the greatest benefit from SRM, you also need a practical framework for application in day-to-day flying. One such approach involves regular evaluation of: *Plan, Plane, Pilot, Passengers,* and *Programming*.

The point of the 5P approach is not to memorize yet another aviation mnemonic. You might simply write these words on your kneeboard, or add a reference to 5Ps to your checklist for key decision points during the flight. These include preflight, pre-takeoff, cruise, pre-descent, and just prior to the final approach fix or, for VFR operations, just prior to entering the traffic pattern.

Items to consider in association with the 5Ps might include the following:

Plan

The plan includes the basic elements of cross-country planning: weather, route, fuel, current publications, etc. The plan also includes all the events that surround the flight and allow the pilot to accomplish the mission. The pilot should review and update the plan at regular intervals in the flight, bearing in mind that any of the factors in the original plan can change at any time.

Plane

The plane includes the airframe, systems, and equipment, including avionics. The pilot should be proficient in the use of all installed equipment as well as familiar with the aircraft/equipment's performance characteristics and limitations. As the flight proceeds, the pilot should monitor the aircraft's systems and instruments in order to detect any abnormal indications at the earliest opportunity.

Continued on Next Page

Pilot

The pilot needs to pass the traditional "IMSAFE" checklist (see below). This part of the 5P process helps a pilot identify and mitigate physiological hazards at all stages of the flight.

Passengers

The passengers can be a great help to the pilot by performing tasks such as those listed earlier. However, passenger needs — e.g., physiological discomfort, anxiety about the flight, or desire to reach the destination — can create potentially dangerous distractions. If the passenger is a pilot, it is also important to establish who is doing what. The 5P approach reminds the pilot-in-command to consider and account for these factors.

Programming

The programming can refer to both panel-mounted and hand-held equipment. Today's electronic instrument displays, moving map navigators, and autopilots can reduce pilot workload and increase pilot situational awareness. However, the task of programming or operating both installed and handheld equipment (e.g., tablets) can create a serious distraction from other flight duties. This part of the 5P approach reminds the pilot to mitigate this risk by having a thorough understanding of the equipment long before takeoff, and by planning in advance when and where the programming for approaches, route changes, and airport information gathering should be accomplished, as well as times it should not be attempted.

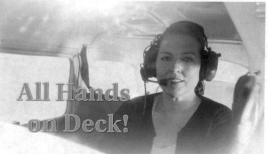

Managing the Mission with a Crew of Just You

Whatever SRM approach you choose, use it consistently and remember that solid SRM skills can significantly enhance the safety of "crew of you" flights.

I'M SAFE Checklist

- **Illness:** Do I have any symptom?
- **Medication:** Have I been taking prescription or over-the-counter drugs?
- **Stress:** Am I under psychological pressure from the job? Am I worried about financial matters, health problems, or family discord?
- **Alcohol:** Have I been drinking within 8 hours?
- **Fatigue:** Am I tired and not adequately rested?
- **Emotion:** Am I emotionally upset?

Resources

- **FAA Risk Management Handbook (Chapter 6)**
  http://1.usa.gov/1Lyumk4
- **Advisory Circular 120-51E,** *Crew Resource Management Training*
  http://go.usa.gov/ZECw

FAST
Federal Aviation Administration
SAFETY TEAM

Appendix IV

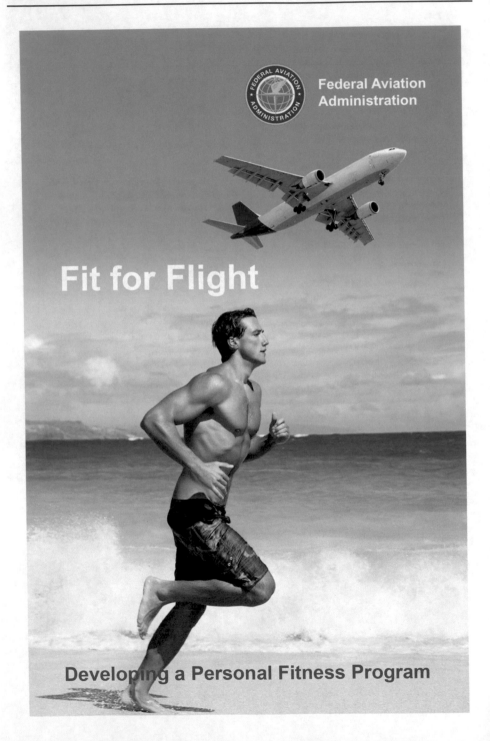

The purpose of this brochure is to provide you with basic guidelines for developing a balanced physical fitness program and customizing a workout to fit your needs. We recommend that you consult a physician before starting any type of physical fitness program. Additionally, an exercise physiologist or professional trainer can help you personalize a specific fitness program.

Benefits of Being Physically Fit

"Use it or lose it!" That old saying not only relates to certain flying skills but also to the human body. Muscles that aren't used tend to atrophy and weaken. To keep muscles and the cardiovascular system working at their optimum levels, they must be stimulated and utilized. Being more physically fit will generally make you look and feel better. Additionally, people that carry too much weight or are bordering on obesity often encounter many health-related problems, ranging from chronic backaches to advanced cardiovascular disease. Finally, a high level of personal fitness can help you to cope with the various emotional and physical stressors that are encountered in the flight environment.

Get a Physical

Before starting a physical fitness program, it is very important that you get a thorough physical examination. Make sure that you tell your medical professional of your intentions to start a fitness program and get some guidance. Also, it would be a good idea to consult with your AME (aviation medical examiner). These professionals can help to tailor a program that addresses the demands of the flight environment.

A Change in Lifestyle

Always keep in mind that becoming fit requires a lifestyle change: adjusting your diet, eating the appropriate types of food with ideal portions, deciding to walk a short trip rather than to drive it, taking the stairs instead of the elevator. These all require a different frame of mind and a change in your daily routine. That, in itself, can be a stressor. Your body will be tasking muscles and systems more than ever. With the accompanying muscle soreness and fatigue, many get discouraged and simply give up. Start out slow. Gradually increase the intensity of your program as your body adjusts to this new lifestyle. But...don't quit!

Basic Components of a Fitness Program
An effective fitness program includes the following:
- Warm-up
- Flexibility and stretching
- Aerobic conditioning
- Anaerobic conditioning
- Cool-down and stretching

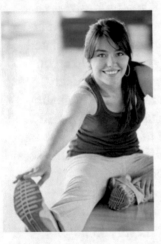

The Warm-Up and Stretch
The warm-up is an essential part of your workout. It should be adjusted to meet the needs of the type of exercise you plan to perform. Warming your muscles gives the body a chance to deliver plenty of nutrient-rich blood to areas about to be exercised and lubricates the joints. The second part of the warm-up process should include stretching. Its purpose is to increase and maintain muscle flexibility by increasing blood flow to the muscles. Stretching should never overextend the muscle or cause it to burn. With the increase in flexibility and range of movement, stretching decreases the risk of injury.

Aerobic (Cardio) Conditioning
Your workout should then involve an aerobic (better known as cardio) activity. Aerobic exercise is any activity that uses large muscle groups, can be maintained continuously, and is rhythmic in nature. The exercise tasks the heart and lungs, causing them to work harder than when at rest.

Some examples of aerobic activities:
- Bicycling (on a stationary bike, if preferred)
- Fitness walking (treadmill, if preferred)
- Jumping rope

- Running or jogging (treadmill, if preferred)
- Stair climbing (or Stairmaster, if preferred)
- Swimming
- Organized sports like softball, basketball, volleyball, racquetball

Anaerobic (Resistance) Conditioning

The effectiveness of your workout would be greatly diminished if it didn't include some type of anaerobic, or resistance training, as a basic component. This type of training tasks a particular muscle or muscle group to increase its strength and/or tone. Exercises can be done by using free-weights, resistance machines, and resistance bands. While free-weights have the advantage of being the most effective, they also have the disadvantage of being less safe. Machines are inherently safer but are less effective. No matter which route you choose, you should always consult a Certified Fitness Professional for proper instruction on equipment use and customizing a "lifting program" tailored to your specific needs. Some examples of anaerobic exercise are:

- Squat
- Bench Press
- Deadlift
- Bicep Curl
- Triceps Extension
- Military Press
- Row

Cool-Down and Stretch

This is the finishing touch to your workout, a very important part of an overall workout because it keeps the body active, prevents the blood from pooling in your extremities, and flushes the muscles of lactic acid. The cool-down should be performed at a low-intensity of effort, starting with the major muscle groups. Similar to the start of our workout, the cool-down period should also involve stretching. A good cool-down with stretching also helps to limit muscle soreness later.

Nutritional Considerations

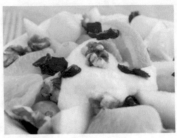

Proper nutrition, fluid intake, rest, and recuperation are important factors for any healthy lifestyle. As your exercise routine increases, these components become more important, as the body needs adequate supplies of these ingredients to function properly. Eating well-balanced meals helps to replenish the nutritional needs of muscles and aids in recuperating from your workouts. A well-balanced meal involves being aware of your intake—especially proteins, carbohydrates, and fats. Most individuals involved in a moderate exercise lifestyle benefit from a diet consisting of meals that are 50-55% complex carbohydrates, 15–20% protein, and 25–35% fat. However, the carbohydrate and protein intake percentages should change, depending on the purpose of your exercise program.

Dehydration is a problem for most people, especially when they begin a fitness program. Exercisers should drink more water than ever before to avoid fatigue and cramping. The average, sedentary person needs two to four quarts of water every 24 hours for normal functioning. Depending on the workout, the weather, and your physical condition, your water intake will need to be increased.

Your Exercise Program

- Can be very simple or very complex in nature
- Should fit your personal needs, lifestyle, and personality
- Should start slowly and build as you adapt; the old sports adage, "no pain, no gain," can be very harmful and should by replaced by "in all things, moderation."

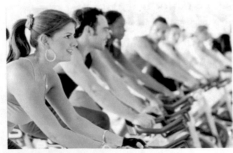

Just Do It!

Physical fitness is a proven component of a long and healthy life. Physical fitness can also prolong your aviation activities by helping you pass your flight physicals.

MEDICAL FACTS FOR PILOTS
Publication No. AM-400/09/2

Written by:
J.R. Brown
Federal Aviation Administration
Civil Aerospace Medical Institute

To request copies of this brochure, contact:
FAA Civil Aerospace Medical Institute
Shipping Clerk, AAM-400
P.O. Box 25082
Oklahoma City, OK 73125
(405) 954-4831

Physiological Training Classes for Pilots

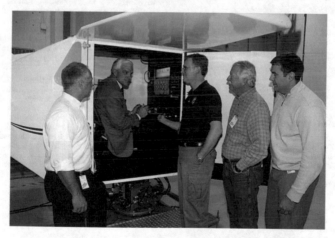

If you are interested in taking a one-day aviation physiological training course with altitude chamber and vertigo demonstrations or a one-day survival course, learn about how to sign up for these courses that are offered at 14 locations across the U.S. by visiting this FAA Web site:
www.faa.gov/pilots/training/airman_education/aerospace_physiology/index.cfm

Appendix V

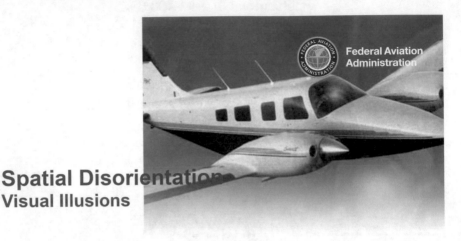

Spatial Disorientation
Visual Illusions

SPATIAL DISORIENTATION:
Seeing Is Not Believing

Spatial Orientation
Our natural ability to maintain our body orientation and/ or posture in relation to the surrounding environment at rest and during motion. Genetically speaking, humans are designed to maintain spatial orientation on the ground. The flight environment is hostile and unfamiliar to the human body; it creates sensory conflicts and illusions that make spatial orientation difficult, and, in some cases, even impossible to achieve. Statistics show that between 5 to 10% of all general aviation accidents can be attributed to spatial disorientation, and 90% of these accidents are fatal.

Spatial Orientation on the Ground
Good spatial orientation on the ground relies on the effective perception, integration, and interpretation of visual, vestibular (organs of equilibrium located in the inner ear), and proprioceptive (receptors located in the skin, muscles, tendons, and joints) sensory information. Changes in linear acceleration, angular acceleration, and gravity are detected by the vestibular system and the proprioceptive receptors, and then compared in the brain with visual information (Figure 1).

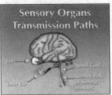

Figure 1

Spatial Orientation In Flight
Spatial orientation in flight is sometimes difficult to achieve because the various types of sensory stimuli (visual, vestibular, and proprioceptive) vary in magnitude, direction, and frequency. Any differences or discrepancies between visual, vestibular, and proprioceptive sensory inputs result in a "sensory mismatch" that can produce illusions and lead to spatial disorientation.

Vision and Spatial Orientation
Visual references provide the most important sensory information to maintain spatial orientation on the ground and during flight, especially when the body and/or the environment are in motion. Even birds, reputable flyers, are unable to maintain spatial orientation and fly safely when deprived of vision (due to clouds or fog). Only bats have developed the ability to fly without vision by replacing their vision with auditory echolocation. So, it should not be any surprise to us that, when we fly under conditions of limited visibility, we have problems maintaining spatial orientation.

Central Vision
Central vision, also known as foveal vision, is involved with the identification of objects and the perception of colors. During instrument flight rules (IFR) flights, central vision allows pilots to acquire information from the flight instruments that is processed by the brain to provide orientational information. During visual flight rules (VFR) flights, central vision allows pilots to acquire external information (monocular and binocular) to make judgments of distance, speed, and depth.

Peripheral Vision

Peripheral vision, also known as ambient vision, is involved with the perception of movement (self and surrounding environment) and provides peripheral reference cues to maintain spatial orientation. This capability enables orientation independent from central vision, and that is why we can walk while reading. With peripheral vision, motion of the surrounding environment produces a perception of self-motion even if we are standing or sitting still.

Visual References

Visual references that provide information about distance, speed, and depth of visualized objects include:

- Comparative size of known objects at different distances.

- Comparative form or shape of known objects at different distances.

- Relative velocity of images moving across the retina. Nearby objects are perceived as moving faster than distant objects.

- Interposition of known objects. One object placed in front of another is perceived as being closer to the observer.

- Varying texture or contrast of known objects at different distances. Object detail and contrast are lost with distance.

- Differences in illumination perspective of objects due to light and shadows.

- Differences in aerial perspective of visualized objects. More distant objects are seen as bluish and blurry.

The flight attitude of an airplane is generally determined by the pilot's visual reference to the natural horizon. When the natural horizon is obscured, attitude can sometimes be maintained by visual reference to the surface below. If neither horizon nor surface visual references exist, the airplane's attitude can only be determined by artificial means such as an attitude indicator or other flight instruments. Surface references or the natural horizon may at times become obscured by smoke, fog, smog, haze, dust, ice particles, or other phenomena, although visibility may be above VFR minimums. This is especially true at airports located adjacent to large bodies of water or sparsely populated areas, where few, if any, surface references are available. Lack of horizon or surface reference is common on over-water flights, at night, or in low visibility conditions.

Visual Illusions

Visual illusions are familiar to most of us. As children, we learned that railroad tracks—contrary to what our eyes showed us—don't come to a point at the horizon. Even under conditions of good visibility, you can experience visual illusions including:

Aerial Perspective Illusions may make you change (increase or decrease) the slope of your final approach. They are caused by runways with different widths, upsloping or downsloping runways, and upsloping or downsloping final approach terrain.

Pilots learn to recognize a normal final approach by developing and recalling a mental image of the expected relationship between the length and the width of an average runway, such as that exemplified in Figure 2.

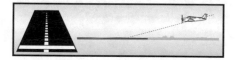

A final approach over a flat terrain with an **upsloping runway** may produce the visual illusion of a high-altitude final approach. If you believe this illusion, you may respond by pitching the aircraft nose down to decrease the altitude, which, if performed too close to the ground, may result in an accident (Figure 3).

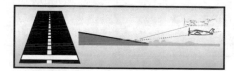

A final approach over a flat terrain with a **downsloping runway** may produce the visual illusion of a low-altitude final approach. If you believe this illusion, you may respond by pitching the aircraft nose up to increase the altitude, which may result in a low-altitude stall or missed approach (Figure 4).

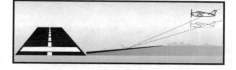

A final approach over an **upsloping terrain** with a flat runway may produce the visual illusion that the aircraft is higher than it actually is. If you believe this illusion, you may respond by pitching the aircraft nose-down to decrease the altitude, resulting in a lower approach. This may result in landing short or flaring short of the runway and risking a low-altitude stall. Pitching the aircraft nose-down will result in a low, dragged-in approach. If power settings are not adjusted, you may find yourself short of the runway, needing to add power to extend your flare. If you do not compensate with power, you will land short or stall short of the runway (Figure 5).

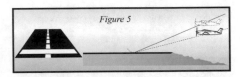

Figure 5

A final approach over a **downsloping terrain** with a flat runway may produce the visual illusion that the aircraft is lower than it actually is. If you believe this illusion, you may respond by pitching the aircraft's nose up to gain altitude. If this happens, you will land further down the runway than you intended (Figure 6).

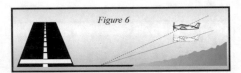

Figure 6

A final approach to an **unusually narrow** runway or an **unusually long** runway may produce the visual illusion of being too high. If you believe this illusion, you may pitch the aircraft's nose down to lose altitude. If this happens too close to the ground, you may land short of the runway and cause an accident (Figure 7).

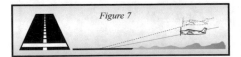

Figure 7

A final approach to an **unusually wide runway** may produce the visual illusion of being lower than you actually are. If you believe this illusion, you may respond by pitching the aircraft's nose up to gain altitude, which may result in a low-altitude stall or missed approach (Figure 8).

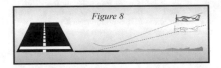

Figure 8

A Black-Hole Approach Illusion can happen during a final approach at night (no stars or moonlight) over water or unlighted terrain to a lighted runway beyond which the horizon is not visible. In the example shown in Figure 9, when peripheral visual cues are not available to help you orient yourself relative to the earth, you may have the illusion of being upright and may perceive the runway to be tilted left and upsloping. However, with the horizon visible (Figure 10) you can easily orient yourself correctly using your central vision.

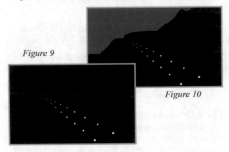

Figure 9

Figure 10

A particularly hazardous black-hole illusion involves approaching a runway under conditions with no lights before the runway and with city lights or rising terrain beyond the runway. Those conditions may produce the visual illusion of a high-altitude final approach. If you believe this illusion you may respond by lowering your approach slope (Figure 11).

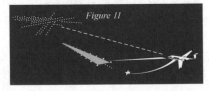

Figure 11

The **Autokinetic Illusion** gives you the impression that a stationary object is moving in front of the airplane's path; it is caused by staring at a fixed single point of light (ground light or a star) in a totally dark and featureless background. This illusion can cause a misperception that such a light is on a collision course with your aircraft (Figure 12).

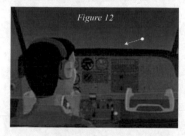

Figure 12

False Visual Reference Illusions may cause you to orient your aircraft in relation to a false horizon; these illusions are caused by flying over a banked cloud, night flying over featureless terrain with ground lights that are indistinguishable from a dark sky with stars, or night flying over a featureless terrain with a clearly defined pattern of ground lights and a dark, starless sky (Figure 13).

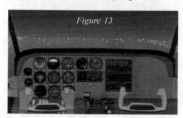

Figure 13

Vection Illusion: A common example is when you are stopped at a traffic light in your car and the car next to you edges forward. Your brain interprets this peripheral visual information as though you are moving backwards and makes you apply additional pressure to the brakes. A similar illusion can happen while taxiing an aircraft (Figure 14).

Figure 14

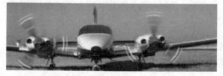

How to Prevent Spatial Disorientation

• Take the opportunity to personally experience sensory illusions in a Barany chair, a Vertigon, a GYRO, or a Virtual Reality Spatial Disorientation Demonstrator (VRSDD). By experiencing sensory illusions first-hand (on the ground), pilots are better prepared to recognize a sensory illusion when it happens during flight and to take immediate and appropriate action. The Aerospace Medical Education Division of the FAA Civil Aerospace Medical Institute offers spatial disorientation demonstrations with the GYRO and the VRSDD in Oklahoma City and at all of the major airshows in the continental U.S.

• Obtain training and maintain your proficiency in aircraft control by reference to instruments.

• When flying at night or in reduced visibility, use and rely on your flight instruments.

• Study and become familiar with unique geographical conditions where flight is intended.

• Do not attempt visual flight when there is a possibility of being trapped in deteriorating weather.

• If you experience a visual illusion during flight (most pilots do at one time or another), have confidence in your instruments and ignore all conflicting signals your body gives you. Accidents usually happen as a result of a pilot's indecision to rely on the instruments.

• If you are one of two pilots in an aircraft and you begin to experience a visual illusion, transfer control of the aircraft to the other pilot, since pilots seldom experience visual illusions at the same time.

• By being knowledgeable, relying on experience, and trusting your instruments, you will be contributing to keeping the skies safe for everyone.

Medical Facts for Pilots

Publication AM-400-00/1 (rev. 2/11)
Revised by: Melchor J. Antuñano, M.D.
FAA Civil Aerospace Medical Institute

To request copies, contact:
FAA Civil Aerospace Medical Institute
Shipping Clerk, AAM-400
P.O. Box 25082 Oklahoma City, OK 73125
(405) 954-4831
A complete list of pilot safety brochures
is on the FAA Web site:
www.faa.gov/pilots/safety/pilotsafetybrochures/

Appendix VI

ICAO LANGUAGE PROFICIENCY REQUIREMENTS IMPLEMENTATION

RECOMMENDED ACTION PLAN

Note: State – national legal and/or regulatory authority responsible for adoption and implementation of ICAO Standards (Annex 1).
ANSP (Air Navigation Service Provider) – organization or entity responsible for the provision of air traffic services (Annex 11).
AO (Airline Operator) – airline or the company responsible for the flight operations (Annex 6).

N	ACTIVITY	RESPONSIBLE BODY /DATE	REMARKS
	Phase 1: Actions to reach Level 4 proficiency		
1.	Ensure all stakeholders (pilots, controllers, language teachers, regulators etc.) are familiar with the ICAO language proficiency requirements.	States, ANSPs, AOs. *As soon as possible in case States have failed to do it until now*	Conduct workshops, seminars, meetings at national and regional level.
2.	Adopt/incorporate the ICAO language proficiency requirements (Amendment 164 to Annex 1) into national legislation.	States *As soon as possible in case States have failed to adopt them until now*	
3.	Nominate contact person(s) within States, airlines and ANSPs to be responsible for coordination of matters at the national level dealing with the implementation of the ICAO language proficiency requirements.	States, ANSPs, AOs. *As soon as possible in case States have failed to do it until now*	
4.	Establish a plan to coordinate administrative and training matters (entry testing, number of personnel to be trained, training centres, duration of training, etc.).	States, ANSPs, AOs. *As soon as possible in case States have failed to do it until now*	
5	Develop/select test(s) to meet ICAO language proficiency requirements.	States, ANSPs, AOs. *As soon as possible*	Ensure test meets requirements of the ICAO Doc 9835. *See Note 1 below the table*
6.	For the selected test(s): select and train personnel to administer, conduct and rate the test(s) • determine the minimum level of proficiency for testing personnel; • provide training in the specialist functions required of testing; and • establish a programme of accreditation for selected testing personnel.	States, ANSPs, AOs *As soon as possible once a test(s) has(have) been selected, but not later than 05 March 2008*	*See Note 2 below the table for desired profiles and requirements*
7.	Obtain certification and/or accreditation of selected test(s) as "an acceptable means of compliance" from national supervisory authority (regulator/civil aviation authority).	States, ANSPs, AOs. *As soon as possible once a test(s) has(have) been selected, but not later than 05 March 2008*	
8.	Assess current language proficiency level of controllers and pilots, according to the ICAO rating scale.	States, ANSPs, AOs. *As soon as possible in case States have failed to do it until now*	Determine magnitude of problem, address individual training needs.

- 2 -

N	ACTIVITY	RESPONSIBLE BODY /DATE	REMARKS
9.	Develop language training packages designed to close the gap between current language proficiency level and ICAO Level 4.	States, ANSPs, AOs, providers of language training. *As soon as possible in case States have failed to do it until now*	Training package includes: plan, syllabus, materials, methods. Language training should be considered in context of job. Note: performance below level 3 will require more general language teaching. Aviation specific language training should be introduced once the ICAO level 3 has been attained.
10.	Assess the financial implications needed to meet ICAO language proficiency requirements. Determine if assistance is required and how it might be obtained.	States, ANSPs, AOs. *As soon as possible in case States have failed to do it until now*	Refer to ICAO Doc 9835 chapter 1.3 for guidance on assistance with training programmes. *See Note 1 below the table*
11.	Identify social issues resulting from implementation of the ICAO language proficiency requirements, and prepare measures to resolve these issues.	States, ANSPs, Aos and social partners. *As soon as possible*	
12.	Familiarise pilots and controllers with the format of the test(s) and procedures for administration of the test.	ANSPs, AOs. *Before testing.*	Organise briefings and make sample tests available for pilots and controllers.
13.	Develop language training package to maintain language proficiency and a schedule of language refresher training.	ANSPs, AOs. *In place before 05 March 2008*	Ensure that current Level 4 is not eroded (could be included in refresher training programmes)
14.	Review recruitment and selection procedures and consider a minimum of at least ICAO level 3 in language proficiency before entry to professional training programmes.	Training establishments, ANSPs, AOs. *Not later than 2007.*	
15.	Implement language awareness programmes to ensure that native and expert speakers of English communicate in a manner that is easily understandable to non-native speakers of English (proficient at ICAO Level 4).	States, AOs, ANSPs *Not later than 05 March 2008*	Applies equally where other languages are used in aeronautical communication
16.	Present preliminary reports to ICAO on progress achieved in preparing for implementation of ICAO language proficiency requirements.	States *2006, 2007.*	
Phase 2: Actions to maintain Level 4 (or higher) proficiency			
17.	Implement testing of pilots and controllers.	States, ANSPs, AOs. *Before 05 March 2008*	
18.	Implement language proficiency maintenance programmes (see item 13 above).	States, ANSPs, AOs. *Before 05 March 2008*	

- 3 -

N	ACTIVITY	RESPONSIBLE BODY /DATE	REMARKS
19.	Extend language testing and training programmes to all pilots and controllers unable to meet the 05 March 2008 deadline.	States, ANSPs, AOs. 2009	
20.	Present a final report to ICAO on implementation of ICAO language proficiency requirements	States *Before 05 March 2008*	

Note 1: ICAO Doc 9835 - Manual on the Implementation of ICAO Language Proficiency Requirement provides guideline material and valuable information on preparing training and testing programmes

Note 2: Suggested profiles for personnel to administer, conduct and rate tests:

Rater - *a person with the English language level proficiency and experience in aviation adequate to evaluate all levers and elements of the ICAO Language Proficiency Rating Scale.*

Tester/Interlocutor - *a person with the English language level proficiency and experience in aviation adequate to conduct the selected test (tests).*

Administrator – *a person familiar with the preparation and conduct of tests/examinations e.g. logistics, security, candidate briefing (could be any of above persons).*

– END –

Appendix VII

Pilot Category	Overview	Suggested Training Requirements & Outcomes	Suggested Duration	Competencies
E	Entry phase. The candidate is not yet type rated and may not necessarily have multi-crew or practical IFR experience.	1. Completed pre-CBT simulator evaluation. 2. Technical Ground School. 3. All aircraft systems and flying training are to be conducted on either the aircraft, or combination of aircraft and simulator. 4. Instrument rating conducted on type. 5. CRM training. 6. Emergency Procedures training (including oxygen use, emergency and life-saving equipment, evacuation procedures, aircraft and passenger control/safety briefing and security training). 7. Operator Proficiency Check: clearance to progress to Cat D.	1. Defined sequences with simplified aircraft configurations and power settings. 2. Technical ground school program (includes FMS training if applicable) + initial flying training with TRI/TRE, including initial aircraft endorsement. Technical, operational, Flight Manual review, Operations Manual review, Dangerous Goods awareness. 3. Approximately 35 hours instrument time with TRI/TRE (may all be in simulator). Defined training syllabus—normally 7 to 8 simulator sessions of 4 hours plus final assessment. 4. Conducted in the simulator 5. CRM 6. Emergency Procedures 7. Minimum of two (2) hours, with TRI/TRE. May be conducted in simulator.	Candidate must hold as a minimum: a CPL (A) licence with 1500 hours total time, 500 multi-engine hours, 100 hours command time and ATPL theory at commencement. On completion, the candidate will have a type rating and Instrument rating, together with any additional legislative or contractual requirements.
D	Line training phase commences.	1. Line operations. Exposure to a representative sample of routes and instrument approaches as both Pilot Flying (PF) and Pilot Not Flying (PNF). Shall include night flying. 2. Discussions with LTC to include abnormal and emergency operations and performance related issues. 3. Line Check: clearance to progress to Cat C.	1. Focus on routine operations including exposure to a representative sample of routes and instrument approaches from copilot seat. A minimum of 3 of each type of instrument approach shall be flow as both PF and PNF. Minimum of 20 sectors with LTC. A sector shall be regarded as a flight between the departure and destination airfields, where all normal checklists are employed. 2. Normally conducted in cruise flight, but may be accomplished 1:1 with trainee and LTC in classroom environment. 3. With TR/TRE. 4 sectors, involving both administrative and flying duties as PF and PNF.	Consistent, safe handling. Cleared to line as a competent copilot.

C	Supervised consolidation flying.	1. Supervised line flying. 2. Line Check: clearance to progress to Cat B.	1. Right hand seat flying only with LTC to syllabus defined minimum criteria. Must cover all normal, abnormal and emergency considerations and include client specific requirements. Recommended minimum time 200 hours. 2. With TRI/TRE. 4 sectors, involving both administrative and flying duties as PF and PNF.	Perform copilot duties with minimal supervision. Sound application and understanding of all normal and emergency operations.
B	Copilot line flying phase.	1. Line flying with indirect supervision. 2. Will include 6-month simulator Proficiency Check. 3. Category A Upgrade Check: clearance to progress to ICUS phase.	1. 500 hours or six months on type (assumes flight hours accrued at 1000 hours per annum): may be crewed with line captains. During this phase, the line captain is to possess at least 500 in command on the aircraft type. 2. 2 x 4 hour simulator sessions covering training elements and the equivalent of IRR. Conducted by TRI/TRE. 3. With TRI/TRE. Will include both line and simulator flying.	Consistent, safe handling in all operational conditions. High level of theoretical and technical knowledge. Manages complex emergencies. Employs CRM skillset throughout.
A	Command Endorsement phase.	1. Command Upgrade course consisting of the following minimum elements: Legal aspects of Command, Regulatory Requirements, Aircraft erformance, Supervision of crew (on and off duty), Technical Ground School refresher, Command CRM, Leadership and Interpersonal Skills required for command, Effective communication, Supervision of flying by First Officers and Effective decision making. 2. LHS flying in simulator. All sessions with designated ICUS training captain. 3. Command upgrade assessment: clearance to progress to command phase.	1. Conducted by Head of Check and Training or delegate. 2. Minimum of 5 x 4 hour sessions covering all aspects of aircraft operation in normal and emergency operations. 3. With TRI/TRE: conducted in a simulator.	Candidate must possess ATPL (A) theory subjects. Command standard in normal and emergency theory, skill and multi-crew procedures.

| Command Upgrade | Command upgrade phase. | Command Upgrade. Suggested requirements:

1. Not less than 50 sectors on type.

2. Minimum of 40 hours of ICUS line flying.

3. Line check (aircraft) | 1. Time must be accrued in aircraft. May consist of time as co-pilot and ICUS.

2. Flown with ICUS training captain as both PF and PNF. Must include consideration of co-pilot supervision throughout the range of flight operations.

3. Line check with TRE. | Command standard in normal and emergency theory, skill and multi-crew procedures.

Successfully completed all Training and Checking Manual competencies.

Completed all instrument rating requirements, including recency, to command standard. |

Index

Printed in the United States
By Bookmasters